HIATAL HERNIA SYNDROME

MANY SYMPTOMS | ONE CAUSE

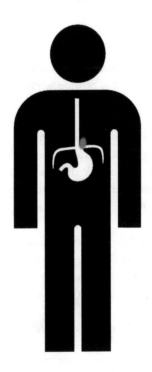

Drs. Vikki & Rick Petersen
DC, CCN, IFMCP

ROOT CAUSE PUBLISHING

Hiatal Hernia Syndrome: Many Symptoms, One Cause
by Drs. Vikki and Rick Petersen, DC, CCN, IFMCP
Published by Root Cause Publishing, 20398
Blauer Drive, Saratoga, CA 95070

Book jacket design and anatomical watercolors by Erica Falke.

This publication contains the opinions and ideas of its
authors. It is intended to provide helpful and informative
material on the subjects addressed in the publication.

For more information, please visit *www.RootCauseMedicalClinics.com*

ISBN 978-0-9822711-4-8
ISBN 978-0-9822711-5-5 (ebook)

Library of Congress Control Cataloging-in-Publication Data is available.

This book is dedicated to those tenacious individuals who are willing to fight for their health and will not give up until they find the true root cause underlying their symptoms.

We wrote this for those who refuse to "put up" with feeling sick.

If you are tenacious and question conventional medical "authority" when what you are told makes no sense to you, this book, and our approach, is what you have been looking for.

Functional Medicine – and our unique version of it, Root Cause Medicine – is for you if you dislike consuming dangerous medications and rather believe in your body's inherent ability to heal with the assistance of a personalized, natural treatment method.

This book is for those who have been told they are "fine" when they in fact feel terrible, and for those who have been told "your symptoms are all in your head."

The truth is you are not making it up, your symptoms are real and in this book you will find the answers you have been looking for.

Never give up on yourself – it is your health, your life and your future hopes and dreams. Fight for yourself and know we are here to assist you in any way we can.

To regaining your best health,

Drs. Vikki and Rick Petersen, DC, CCN, IFMCP

CONTENTS

CHAPTER 1

INTRODUCTION TO ROOT CAUSE MEDICINE

Functional medicine, or what we call Root Cause Medicine, is a methodology of looking at the body as a whole. It appreciates that no part of your body works in a vacuum and that all your organs and systems affect one another.

Root Cause Medicine further appreciates that your body's ability to heal itself is rather amazing. It is a strong machine with "parts" designed to last 120 years. That is correct: your body's organs have a life expectancy of 120 years when you treat them properly.

When the body is not functioning optimally it is because an excessive number of burdens have overwhelmed your body, and its ability to heal itself has become compromised.

Your body wants to let you know it has become overwhelmed by the burdens and it does so by giving you symptoms.

Symptoms are your body's only way of letting you know that it has become overburdened to such a degree that its ability to heal itself has been overwhelmed. Symptoms are your body's "text message" system to you, its only means of communicating to you that it needs help.

In our country, do you think conventional medicine tends to address the symptom or the underlying root cause of the symptom? We have asked hundreds of people this question during lectures across Silicon Valley and beyond. What we have found is that the majority agree: our medical system is primarily symptom oriented. Conventional medicine directs itself toward managing your symptoms, typically with drugs.

It is a problem for many reasons.

First, the approach is not respectful of your body's ability to heal itself.

Second, it introduces dangerous chemicals that overwhelm the function of your body and cause dangerous side effects. If you have acid reflux, here is an antacid. (We will be discussing the dangers of antacids later.) If you have a headache, here is a pain reliever. If you have high blood pressure, here is another drug; often two are prescribed.

Let us take up the last example, the very common condition of high blood pressure. Discussing it will help differentiate the conventional medicine approach from that of Root Cause Medicine.

If you arrived at my clinic and you unknowingly had excessively high blood pressure, we would often prescribe for you a medication in the same way any conventional medicine clinic would. After all, we do not want you to suffer a stroke or some other life-threatening condition. (Keep in mind we are using the example of excessively high blood pressure here.)

When you are put on blood pressure medication by a conventional doctor, you are typically told the medication is for life. You may later be prescribed a higher dose, you may one day change to a different medication, or perhaps add an additional one because the medication loses efficacy. The medications may change, but you are told you will be on some type of blood pressure medication for the rest of your life.

It is worth noting that while chronically elevated blood pressure can damage your kidneys, kidney disease is one side effect of commonly used blood pressure medications. You are told that you need to lower your blood pressure to "protect" your kidneys, but you are not typically told of the risk to those very organs that your medication causes.

Diuretics, or water pills, are associated with a risk of acute kidney injury.

ACE inhibitors (drugs such as lisinopril and most drugs ending with "-il") are prescribed for high blood pressure and heart failure, but they do pose a risk of kidney damage, especially if you are dehydrated (a common condition for Americans).

Once your kidneys fail, dialysis is prescribed. A life of dialysis treatments several times per week is an awful experience.

What if you could normalize your blood pressure without the use of dangerous drugs?

In Root Cause Medicine we take a very different approach from the conventional "life sentence" of medication. We may put you on a drug temporarily to stabilize you if your blood pressure is dangerously high, but the difference is that we do not stop there. We get to work identifying the underlying root cause.

Why is your body creating high blood pressure?

Your body always has a reason for the symptoms it is creating. It is our job to discover what that reason is, and we do not give up until we find it.

Our tenacity comes from the knowledge that there *is* a reason, a root cause. Our tenacity further comes from thirty years of experience and a high success rate that has taught us not to give up until we find it. We know that once we unburden your body enough, it will heal.

And yes, getting our patients to the point they can be safely weaned off their blood pressure medication – because we have identified and successfully treated the true underlying root cause – is something we do regularly.

We have a large armamentarium: testing which allows us to find the answers we need, and tools to treat the root causes we identify.

Once we find the underlying root cause and treat it, your body is unburdened and can heal. We love restoring function to the human body and weaning patients off drugs; it is in fact one of our specialties.

When the body no longer requires the medication, not only are you no longer at risk of dangerous side effects, you know you have restored function and your body is functioning correctly on its own, as it was designed to.

Hopefully, this explains why we feel comfortable in the role of identifying the root cause of a variety of health care complaints and why we often achieve success where other practitioners have failed.

We are very comfortable being the "last resort" for patients who come to us feeling that they have tried "everything" and been "everywhere." We know we have the tools to achieve success.

We are not magicians and we do require your compliance, but our success rate of eighty-five percent is quite high, and it is something we are proud of.

Now that you understand the underlying principle of Root Cause Medicine, in the next chapter we will discuss how we came to write a book on this particular subject.

CHAPTER 2

WHY WE ARE WRITING THIS BOOK

If you are reading this chapter, please make sure you have first read Chapter 1: Introduction to Root Cause Medicine. It will orient you to what we are about to discuss.

Hiatal Hernia Syndrome (HHS) has now been identified and its treatment protocol developed at Root Cause Medical Clinic. We are not new to "coining" conditions that later become widely accepted. When we wrote the book *The Gluten Effect* in 2009, there was no validation of gluten sensitivity, now often termed 'non-celiac gluten sensitivity.'

Celiac disease, an autoimmune condition, was the one confirmed gluten "disease" at the time. Yet we found ourselves successfully treating patients who were afflicted with neither celiac disease nor a wheat allergy.

The changes in our patients were miraculous. For those suffering from a range of conditions – from seizures to migraines, from IBS-like conditions to anxiety, and from PMS to infertility – the removal of gluten from the diet was incredibly beneficial. This "gluten problem" that was not celiac disease was able to affect every organ system in the human body.

What to call it? We decided to call it gluten sensitivity and wrote an entire book about it. It was an interesting feeling, writing our first book about a problem we had coined the name of, with no validation of its existence.

We could not help it. We knew what we saw at the clinic and we needed to tell the world, or whomever would listen.

It was not until several years later, in 2012, that validation for gluten sensitivity was finally published in the literature of the broader medical community.

So here we are again, needing to tell the world about something it is already aware of on some level, but about which the big picture is entirely missing.

Hiatal Hernia Syndrome encompasses a vast number of seemingly disrelated symptoms, at least twenty in number, that can occur as a result of this syndrome.

While hiatal hernia is a known condition, Hiatal Hernia Syndrome embraces what conventional medicine denies, and that is the connection between hiatal hernia and such symptoms as:

- Heart palpitations
- Chest pain
- Panic attacks
- Anxiety

- Shortness of breath
- Bloating and gas
- Shoulder and arm pain
- Back pain
- Constipation
- And more.

We are writing this book because this syndrome is common.

We are writing this book because too many Americans, and others across the planet, have their lives terribly disrupted (if not ruined) by a syndrome that their conventional doctor does not acknowledge.

We are writing this book because every day in an E.R. and/or Urgent Care facility someone is told they are having a panic attack, when the true cause is actually Hiatal Hernia Syndrome. These patients are put on dangerous psychiatric medications when their problem is completely physical at its root.

We are writing this book because acid reflux and heartburn are treated with dangerous antacids that have horrific side effects.

We are writing this book because you deserve to know the truth.

We hope this information brings you, a friend or loved one the truth that will restore your health, your vitality and your enjoyment of life. It is your life and you deserve to live it to its fullest.

With respect and love,

Drs. Vikki and Rick Petersen, DC, CCN, IFMCP

Founders of Root Cause Medical Clinics

CHAPTER 3

WHAT IS HIATAL HERNIA SYNDROME VS. A HIATAL HERNIA?

We want to begin by defining hiatal hernia.

"Hiatus" means a hole or opening. A "hernia" is a condition in which something is protruding through an opening inappropriately. You may have heard of abdominal or inguinal hernias, where someone's intestines are pushing through an opening or tear in their abdominal muscles.

A hiatal hernia involves your stomach, esophagus, and diaphragm.

First, a little basic anatomy.

Your mouth is connected to your stomach via your esophagus, which is a long tube.

Your stomach lies below your diaphragm, which is a series of strong, flat muscles that contract and relax, allowing you to breathe deeply, getting good oxygen. The diaphragm muscles must move freely up and down to allow for a normal flow of oxygen, but the diaphragm also does a great deal more, which we will discuss later.

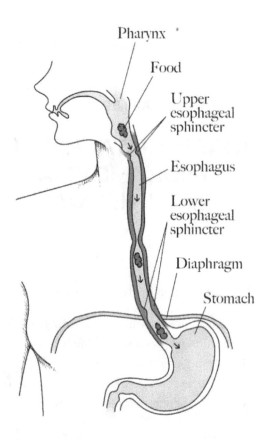

Spoiler alert: A hiatal hernia can result in shortness of breath, panic attacks or heart palpitations, as a result of the diaphragm being unable to move freely.

At the base of your esophagus there is a valve, or sphincter, that opens while you are swallowing, allowing food to move into your stomach. (This is called the lower esophageal sphincter, or LES). When food is not passing down your esophagus, the sphincter closes off, preventing the contents of your stomach from moving in the wrong direction i.e. up into the esophagus.

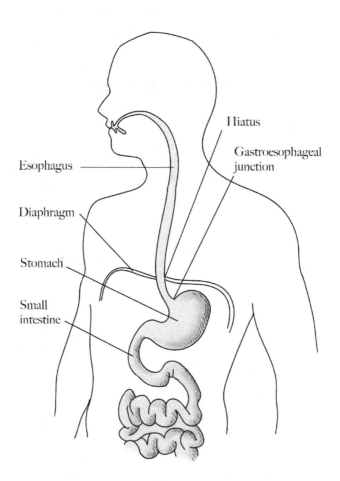

It turns out the tendons of your diaphragm also contribute to the integrity and correct operation of your esophageal sphincter.

When this "wrong direction of stomach contents" occurs, it is called reflux or GERD (gastroesophageal reflux disease). If you have ever experienced heartburn or acid reflux (GERD), you know how it feels when food or acid has moved in the wrong direction, i.e. up into your esophagus from your stomach.

Of course, the more dramatic experience is vomiting. This is a sudden reversal of the contents of your stomach up into your esophagus.

The normal direction is from the top to the bottom: from your mouth, down your esophagus and into the stomach, with the sphincter correctly closing off and preventing any "wrong-directional" flow.

A hiatal hernia, in its classic sense, is when the stomach has pushed up through the esophageal sphincter and is now above your diaphragm.

Normal Stomach   Hiatal Hernia

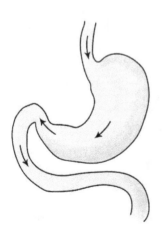
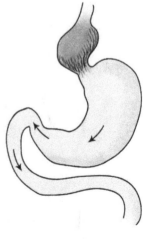

Typically, doctors recommend nothing for treating this condition, other than antacids if GERD or heartburn is present.

In rare circumstances, the stomach has moved up so high that surgery is required – this is a serious and uncommon condition, and not the subject of this book.

There are other types of hiatal hernia that, while considered mild, still cause severe symptoms. We will discuss those later.

HIATAL HERNIA SYNDROME

Hiatal Hernia Syndrome (HHS) is more embracive than just hiatal hernia: it encompasses all the potential contributors to a syndrome able to cause twenty or so different symptoms.

What we are about to say may sound a bit unbelievable to you right now, but it will make sense once you have read the rest of this book.

HHS potentially involves many systems and organs in your body. There is not a "one size fits all" treatment for HHS. Conventional medicine gives antacids and leaves it at that. This is a disservice to you in many ways.

The Root Cause Medical Clinics' treatment of HHS entails a full evaluation of the function (or malfunction) of your:

- Diaphragm integrity
- Stomach
- Liver and gall bladder
- Small and large intestine
- Microbiome (the bacteria within your colon – numbering about thirty-nine trillion – that make up about eighty percent of your immune system)
- Heart function
- Diet, including evaluation of any food sensitivities and overall quality
- Nutrient levels
- Toxicity levels
- Stress hormones
- Sex hormones

- Spinal alignment including neck, ribs, middle and lower back vertebrae
- Muscle balance or imbalance of your neck, torso, lower back, hip and core abdominal muscles
- And more.

Do not be intimidated by this list; it is unlikely you will require intervention in all these areas. But since these are all potential contributors to the problem, it is important to evaluate them. We tailor our programs to each patient individually, and a thorough program requires checking every area of potential malfunction.

It is precisely because the list of potential symptoms is so long that Hiatal Hernia Syndrome can be referred to as 'the great mimic.' Conventional doctors who have no knowledge of the syndrome can be easily led astray, referring their patients to cardiologists, pulmonologists, endocrinologists and psychiatrists. Those of you who have been suffering for a while and seeking help unsuccessfully know exactly what we mean.

There is an upcoming chapter on the anatomy of the diaphragm and hiatal hernia (CHAPTER 6: THE ANATOMY OF HIATAL HERNIA SYNDROME, AN IN-DEPTH LOOK). In it you will see how all the above is interrelated.

In my next chapter you can take a short quiz to see if Hiatal Hernia Syndrome (HHS) explains the cause of some of your health problems.

CHAPTER 4

HIATAL HERNIA SYNDROME QUIZ

D o you have Hiatal Hernia Syndrome? Take this quiz to find out.

Do you suffer with acid reflux or gastroesophageal reflux disease (GERD)? **Note:** Answer "yes" if you've had it but the symptoms are currently "handled" by medication.

1. Have you experienced heart palpitations or a rapid heart rate for no obvious reason?

2. Do you suffer from shortness of breath?

3. Do you have anxiety or panic attacks?

4. Do your symptoms interrupt your sleep?

5. Do you tend towards constipation? (Defined as not easily moving your bowels one to two times per day. If you need to bear down to move your bowels, that is considered constipation.)

6. Do you feel a tightness or pressure in your chest or upper abdomen?

7. Do you suffer from belching, burping, bloating, and/or hiccupping?

8. Do your symptoms worsen with bending over or lying down?

9. Do you experience tightness or pain in your neck, shoulder, upper or middle back?

10. Are you forty years of age or older?

11. Are you overweight, particularly with belly weight?

Add up your "yes" answers. Scoring:

7 or more "yes" answers: It is highly likely you are experiencing some form of Hiatal Hernia Syndrome. Keep reading; this book was written for you!

4 to 6 "yes" answers: It is probable that Hiatal Hernia Syndrome is contributing to the cause of your symptoms. This book should help to shed a lot of light on why you have been suffering.

3 or fewer "yes" answers: While it is not highly likely, do not ignore the symptoms you do have. Keep reading to see if those symptoms could be related to this syndrome.

CHAPTER 5

THE MOST COMMON SYMPTOMS OF HIATAL HERNIA SYNDROME

How would you know if Hiatal Hernia Syndrome (HHS) is affecting you? There are many varied symptoms potentially associated with HHS. We will list them here, and we will go into more specifics on each one below.

Common symptoms include:

1. Heartburn, acid reflux or GERD

2. Trouble swallowing or a constriction in your throat

3. Tightness or pressure in your chest

4. Shortness of breath

5. Heart palpitations

6. Anxiety

7. Panic attacks

8. Light-headedness or dizziness

9. Tingling in hands or feet

10. Chest pain

11. Neck pain or tightness

12. Constipation

13. Bloating or pain in your abdomen

14. Burping

15. Worsening of symptoms with bending over

16. Trouble sleeping, or symptoms worsen when lying down

17. Fatigue

Despite the long list of symptoms, we find a relatively small number of underlying (root) causes.

The following two causes are almost always present:

- imbalance in the functioning of the diaphragm, and
- malfunctioning of the digestive tract.

Let us look at some of the most common symptoms and why they occur.

HEARTBURN AND GERD

Heartburn, acid reflux, or gastroesophageal reflux disease (GERD) are quite common with Hiatal Hernia Syndrome. It is estimated that twenty percent of American adults experience one of these symptoms regularly; some experience them daily.

Common does not mean normal however, and it is certainly not normal nor healthy to suffer acid reflux.

When it comes to cause vs. effect, it is of note that while many people with Hiatal Hernia Syndrome suffer heartburn and GERD, not everyone does. Similarly, many of those suffering with acid reflux do not have a hiatal hernia. These do occur independently.

Likely, the factors contributing to acid reflux that also contribute to hernias are the ones that they share. It makes sense and we will be discussing those causative factors below.

Research does confirm an overlap between the two and it certainly aligns with what we see at the clinic.

Hiatal hernia also shares a common link with Crohn's disease, which is a type of inflammatory bowel disease that causes inflammation of your digestive tract.

Why does it occur?

The stomach is designed to be a bag of acid. When food moves down your esophagus into your stomach it passes through a sphincter or valve at the bottom of the esophagus. The valve opens in response to your action of swallowing. Once food has fully passed into the stomach, the valve closes, preventing any "wrong-directional" flow of food or acid. The integrity of your diaphragm also assists in the valve closing properly.

Acid reflux occurs for some when the valve is functioning inappropriately.

This can be the result of your stomach having pushed up above your diaphragm, where it is unable to keep the valve closed.

It can occur if your stomach is in spasm from something you ate and were unable to properly digest, or due to the presence of an infection.

The result is that the contents of your stomach are pushed up into your esophagus. (Food poisoning can be a dramatic example of this when it results in vomiting.)

This can cause pain or burning in your chest, esophagus, and/or throat. It can also cause regurgitated food to come up into your throat, or even into your nose.

More rarely, it can result in excessive saliva production. Some patients feel like they are choking due to this, especially when lying down.

It is of note that some patients experience acid reflux but have no overt symptoms. This is called silent reflux or laryngopharangeal reflux (to break that word down: your larynx houses your vocal cords; your esophagus is the tube connecting your mouth to your stomach). You are unaware of it, but it can still cause damage. Such damage is often found during an endoscopy procedure.

You can have classic acid reflux, with burning or a bitter taste in your mouth, but you may also experience excessive throat clearing, a nagging cough, hoarseness, or a "lump" in your throat. Another symptom that does not typically lend itself to thinking of acid reflux, but is common with this condition, is a sensation of excess throat mucus, postnasal drip, or a sore throat.

Above we mentioned the possibility of an infection causing acid reflux symptoms. Helicobacter pylori (H. pylori as it has come to be known) is a common bacterium you can be exposed to – it is very pervasive in our environment. If your immune system is healthy, it will deal with it on its own, destroying the bacterium before it can multiply. However, if your immune system is compromised, the H. pylori infection can gain a foothold within your stomach.

Controversy remains about the association of GERD and H. pylori infection. We mention it here because at our clinic we do see a strong association: the infection can lead to the development of GERD.

The bacteria of H. pylori produce an enzyme called urease that breaks urea in the stomach down into carbon dioxide and ammonia. This causes bad breath and burping, due to the neutralizing of the hydrochloric acid in your stomach.

Your stomach is a bag of acid for a reason. Hydrochloric acid (stomach acid) performs many functions:

- Digests protein and ionizes minerals for later absorption.
- Acts as an antimicrobial. (Insufficient quantities are associated with more intestinal infections.)
- Stimulates the release of enzymes from your pancreas, which further break down fats and proteins.
- Stimulates the release of bile from your gall bladder. Bile metabolizes or breaks down fat in your small intestine, plus it acts as an antimicrobial, killing bad organisms in the upper small intestine.

Bile also acts as a detergent in your upper bowel – a role too often forgotten – ensuring any inhospitable organisms are eliminated. SIBO (small intestinal bacterial overgrowth) can be a result of poor bile production.

Lack of adequate acid and of proper bile flow also puts you at risk for anemia, thyroid problems, osteoporosis, and autoimmune disease.

And it all ties to having adequate stomach acid.

Hopefully, you are getting a glimmer as to the dangers of antacids, which prevent all these functions from occurring. We discuss these dangers in greater detail in CHAPTER 11: TREATMENT. There are a variety of symptoms associated with acid reflux, some of which may be surprising to you.

Symptoms of heartburn or GERD

- Heartburn (a burning pain in your chest, just behind your breastbone)
- Bitter taste in your mouth, which can be infrequent or often (Patients describe it as a sour liquid in their throat or even regurgitated food.)
- Waking up in the middle of the night coughing or with a feeling of choking
- Feeling more uncomfortable when bending over or lying down
- Bloating after meals, or just generally
- Burping or gassiness after meals
- Nausea
- Dry mouth or throat irritation

- Gum irritation or tenderness, including bleeding
- Bad breath

Severe symptoms

The following is a list of severe symptoms. If you are experiencing any of the following you should consult your doctor.

- Bloody vomiting or black stools (a possible sign of damage to the lining of your esophagus causing bleeding)
- Hiccups that are difficult to stop
- Difficulty swallowing (can be due to a narrowing esophagus)
- Unexpected weight loss
- Hoarseness upon arising or throughout the day
- Chronic coughing or throat irritation

Long-term GERD can cause bleeding ulcers in the esophagus. The ulcers are sores caused by the damage your stomach acid has inflicted on the lining of your esophagus.

An ulcer may bleed, which is painful and can create difficulty swallowing.

It is important to identify if you have an ulcer; they can be treated naturally if identified early. Natural treatment includes dietary changes and identifying if the bacterial infection H. pylori is present (a known cause of stomach ulcers and acid reflux.) Natural nutrition is utilized to kill any bacteria or other organism present, and to heal the ulcer.

We will discuss more treatment options in CHAPTER 11: TREATMENT.

Bleeding can also result in anemia or iron deficiency anemia. As we have just mentioned, hiatal hernias can result in subtle or more severe bleeding due to the irritating acid in the esophagus.

Minor "micro-bleeds" can occur over a long time and result in anemia. More serious conditions, such as vomiting of blood or blood loss in the stool, can also cause anemia.

Larger hiatal hernias are a known risk for blood loss and anemia. A blood test can identify the presence of anemia, but typically other causes will be investigated first, since hiatal hernias often remain undiagnosed.

When anemia is present in post-menopausal women or in men of any age, a hiatal hernia should be tested for. We mention this as it is not typically evaluated for, adding to the list of reasons Hiatal Hernia Syndrome is vastly underdiagnosed.

A savvy gastroenterologist can identify so-called Cameron lesions at the neck of the hiatal hernia. These would be found during endoscopy but unfortunately are often missed.

Iron deficiency anemia can affect the body in a variety of ways. It occurs when there aren't enough red blood cells to transfer hemoglobin around the body. The heart can be particularly affected because hemoglobin deficiency puts stress on the heart, making it more difficult to pump oxygen-carrying blood throughout your body.

Extreme fatigue or weakness, dizziness or light-headedness are common with anemia. So too is chest pain, fast heartbeat, or shortness of breath. Notice how these latter symptoms are also among those associated with Hiatal Hernia Syndrome.

Additional symptoms of anemia, not in common with Hiatal

Hernia Syndrome: cold hands and feet, inflammation or soreness of the tongue, and brittle nails.

If the condition of bleeding becomes too severe, surgery may be necessary to address the complications of any ulcers, stomach bleeding or esophageal strictures.

Long-standing (untreated) acid reflux can result in the development of Barrett's esophagus, a condition which can increase your risk of esophageal cancer.

Asthma is a respiratory condition whereby your bronchi, or airways, are wracked by spasms, resulting in difficulty breathing; it seems completely unrelated to a digestive problem. But asthma and hiatal hernia do have an interrelationship. The reflux so common with Hiatal Hernia Syndrome may cause asthma in multiple ways.

The stomach acid that leaks into the esophagus can create asthma-like symptoms. The refluxed acid irritates the nerve endings in your esophagus and your brain responds to this by sending impulses to your lungs, stimulating the production of mucus in your bronchi. This causes a constriction of your lungs, which mimics asthma symptoms.

Another cause is aspiration: stomach acid can enter your lungs directly when you draw breath. The stomach acid is a foreign material and your lungs' efforts to expel the invading acid mimic asthma symptoms: trouble breathing, tightness of the chest, sneezing and/ or coughing.

Additionally, there is a potential side effect of asthma medication that may trigger GERD. This occurs when the medication causes the esophageal sphincter, not just the bronchi, to relax too much, thereby allowing the contents of your stomach to move up into your esophagus.

Trouble swallowing or a constriction in your throat

Patients describe this issue in several ways:

- Difficulty swallowing
- Food feels trapped or "stuck" in the esophagus
- Throat feels irritated
- A "scraping" sensation when food travels down the esophagus.

The chronic presence of acid in the esophagus can create irritation and inflammation within its walls. The tube is inflamed, so of course food feels like an irritant as it moves down. Over time, this continuous damage can create scar tissue. The scar tissue can continue to build up and may eventually narrow the esophagus, creating what is known as an esophageal stricture.

The long-term irritation by stomach acid can also change the structure of the cells of the lower esophagus, resulting in what is called Barrett's esophagus. Sometimes there are no noticeable symptoms with Barrett's, but because it can increase your risk of esophageal cancer, it needs to be diagnosed and treated.

Because the chronic presence of acid can result in ulcers and even increased risk of cancer, it is imperative to address the true root cause and fully heal your esophagus.

Tightness or pressure in your chest

A tight or constricting feeling in your chest, especially at the bottom of the sternum or chest bone, is caused by pressure built up between your diaphragm and stomach. When your stomach has moved up above the level of the diaphragm, gas can get trapped, causing you to feel increased tightness and pressure. Sometimes this pressure is temporarily relieved by burping.

The constrictive feeling can also be caused by the spasmed diaphragm: it does not move as readily as it should, resulting in a feeling of tightness or pressure.

Shortness of breath

Shortness of breath, difficulty getting a deep breath, or excessive yawning all occur due to the spasmed or elevated diaphragm. Your body is not getting adequate oxygen due to the lack of normal diaphragmatic excursion, or movement. Your body creates one or more of these symptoms to alert you to the insufficient oxygen levels.

Heart palpitations

Heart palpitations can occur because of the pressure of the stomach and diaphragm irritating your vagus nerve. The vagus nerve is a very long cranial nerve, part of the parasympathetic nervous system. It normally works to slow your heart rate.

When the vagus nerve is irritated it can create a variety of symptoms, including heart palpitations.

Large hiatal hernias can actually compress the left atrium of your heart, causing lack of proper blood flow and the potential for atrial fibrillation, discussed below.

Heart palpitations can be quite scary and frequently send patients to the E.R. to rule out a heart attack. There is nothing wrong with making that your first stop – it is certainly better to be in a hospital if you are having a heart attack.

However, if you have already been to the hospital (and perhaps visited a cardiologist) only to be told your heart is fine, you are not alone. Many patients with undiagnosed and untreated hiatal hernia have had this experience on more than one occasion. It does not make your heart palpitations any less real or any less anxiety-inducing – it just means your heart is healthy. It also means that Hiatal Hernia Syndrome needs to be ruled out as a potential cause.

Atrial fibrillation (an irregular, often rapid heart rate that commonly causes poor blood flow) is a known association with hiatal hernia in men and women of all ages. Younger patients (those under the age of fifty-five) diagnosed with hiatal hernia have a risk as much as nineteen percent higher of experiencing atrial fibrillation.

The reflux of acid into the esophagus from the stomach appears to be a trigger for arrhythmia, or the imbalanced rhythm of your heart that is so disconcerting when you feel it.

Along with heart palpitations, arrhythmia is a common presentation of Hiatal Hernia Syndrome in our patients.

Anxiety

Anxiety that comes upon you for no obvious reason can be very disconcerting. The anxiety is very much present, but your environment does not seem to warrant that reaction.

Internally, your body does have a reason. One such reason is the response of a nerve that is affected when you are not breathing freely. In fact, insufficient breath engages a part of your nervous system which makes it impossible for you to relax.

The nerve is called the vagus nerve and in CHAPTER 11: TREATMENT we discuss how the nerve, when malfunctioning, creates not only anxiety but a host of other symptoms and diseases.

Hiatal Hernia Syndrome always involves your diaphragm to some degree. The diaphragm is your breathing muscle: lack of proper function leads to lack of adequate oxygenation. This puts a burden on your nervous system, which is designed to let you know when you don't have enough air flow. The result is that your body creates stress hormones to put you on high alert.

It is not fun to experience the feeling of anxiety, but realize your body is causing your anxiety as a protective response. It wants you to figure out why you are not getting enough oxygen.

It is a problem that is often "treated" with anxiety medications. These medications have a dangerous potential for creating life-threatening side effects. Not to mention they are attempting to address a problem by changing your brain chemicals when the cause of Hiatal Hernia Syndrome has nothing to do with your brain.

Panic attacks

A panic attack is perhaps best described as anxiety on steroids. It is occurring for the reasons we have just described under anxiety, plus it is exacerbated by heart palpitations and chest tightness.

Panic attacks can occur frequently at night when you are lying down, but also at other times of the day.

It is particularly frightening to wake from a deep sleep in a panic, perhaps with heart palpitations or shortness of breath, and have no idea why.

Such events often lead to emergency room visits, where you are told, "You're fine – you're just having a panic attack."

Unfortunately, E.R. visits often end with a prescription for a dangerous psychiatric drug when your problem is physical and digestive at its root – there is no mental disease occurring.

If your scan or X-ray does not show an overt hiatal hernia and doctors have ruled out a heart condition, you will typically be sent home with a pat on the head and a reassurance that you are "fine". Or you will be sent home with anti-anxiety medication. As we have mentioned, psychiatric medications have very dangerous, potentially life-threatening side effects.

Light-headedness or dizziness

Light-headedness can be vasovagal (a temporary drop in blood pressure caused by overactivity of the vagus nerve), or from lack of oxygen.

Many of the symptoms we have been discussing are interrelated. When you are not getting enough oxygen due to Hiatal Hernia Syndrome, you could manifest anxiety, shortness of breath, a panic attack, or you could feel light-headed or dizzy. The vagus nerve that we mentioned in the ANXIETY section can also be creating a feeling of light-headedness or dizziness.

I'm reviewing each of these interrelated symptoms independently because, if for you the overwhelming symptom is light-headedness or dizziness, that's what you're going to be looking for in this book, and we want to ensure you find answers.

When your diaphragm cannot fully move it is almost like someone is sitting on your chest or subtly putting their hands around your neck, reducing the amount of air you can take in. If you cannot freely inhale all the air you want, your nervous system registers this and you can begin to feel light-headed or dizzy.

Tingling in hands or feet

Tingling in the arms, hands, or feet can occur because of the increased stress hormones. Such tingling can occur along with anxiety or a panic attack. We list it separately because some people notice this more than others. The root cause is the same as we have just discussed under anxiety and panic attacks.

Chest pain

Pain in the chest or upper stomach area after eating or bending over is common in Hiatal Hernia Syndrome.

It is caused by the elevated or spasmed diaphragm which is not allowing for the full and natural movement of your ribs and chest cavity.

It can also be caused by an irritated and elevated stomach. Food should be delivered into a relaxed stomach which then secretes acid and churns your food around for about four hours. If the stomach is in spasm or elevated, it cannot do its job efficiently and you can feel discomfort or pressure, including a bloating feeling, a feeling of trapped gas, or a sensation of not digesting properly.

Neck pain or tightness

The nerve that travels to your diaphragm to make it operate correctly is called the phrenic nerve. It originates in your mid-neck and travels to your diaphragm, following a similar course as your vagus nerve in that area of your body.

When any muscle or organ in your body is irritated, it can reflexively cause the area of the spine from which the related nerve emanates to feel discomfort.

In the case of irritation to the diaphragm, its nerve originates in the neck and thereby can create pain or tightness there.

Neck pain or tightness, therefore, can be the cause or the effect of Hiatal Hernia Syndrome.

We see this association often. It is why chiropractic care and physical therapy are an integral part of our treatment regimen.

Constipation

Constipation of a chronic nature – defined as not easily moving your bowels once or twice per day – is a common symptom of many who suffer from Hiatal Hernia Syndrome.

You can suffer constipation from a variety of causes, but it is the presence of chronic constipation and the increased intra-abdominal pressure it causes that aggravates or initiates HHS.

Hiatal Hernia Syndrome is the culmination of several causes, but as we have mentioned, digestive imbalance is very much a root cause of the condition.

Bloating or pain in your abdomen

Bloating is an indication of poor digestion. It can be the cause or the effect of Hiatal Hernia Syndrome. Poor stomach function can be affected by food sensitivities, bacterial infections, or parasites. The use of antacids which diminish the normal acidic milieu of the stomach exacerbate the problem.

Remember, your stomach is designed to be a bag of acid. It is just not supposed to allow acid to travel up into your esophagus.

Burping

Burping is a common symptom of Hiatal Hernia Syndrome. The gas build-up can become quite uncomfortable and often patients experience temporary relief when they can pass the entrapped gas by burping. The relief is only temporary, however.

The diaphragm dictates the normal exchange of air in both inhalation and exhalation. In Hiatal Hernia Syndrome there is an elevation of both the diaphragm and esophageal sphincter, creating an abnormal pressure differential between your chest and abdomen. Air gets "trapped" and gas and pressure build as a result.

Worsening of symptoms with bending over

Symptoms of Hiatal Hernia Syndrome can worsen when bending over, for example when tying your shoes or picking something up from the floor. With this syndrome your stomach and diaphragm already tend to be "riding high." Bending over increases the intra-abdominal pressure, forcing them to move even higher, hence the worsening of your symptoms.

Trouble sleeping, or symptoms worsen when lying down

Symptoms of Hiatal Hernia Syndrome can worsen when you are sleeping or lying down. During the day gravity is helping to pull your stomach and diaphragm downward. Gravity often is not enough to get them into a completely normal position, but when you lie down all help from gravity disappears and symptoms can become more intense as a result.

Fatigue

Fatigue can be caused by a variety of factors. Certainly, the lower oxygen content is one cause. The increased production of stress hormones and digestive imbalance can also be involved. Stress hormones will rob you of adrenaline, and if you are not turning your food into good, absorbable fuel, fatigue will result.

That was a long list. If you see yourself on it and you have been frustrated with a lack of help from your doctor, we are delighted that you are reading this book. Hopefully, you are gaining an understanding of this syndrome and how your symptoms may fit into its description.

The good news is that it can be treated naturally (meaning without drugs) in the vast majority of cases.

The next chapter delves into the anatomy of the diaphragm and how it affects your body from top to bottom, literally. For those of you who like a deeper understanding, this chapter should enlighten you further.

CHAPTER 6

THE ANATOMY OF HIATAL HERNIA SYNDROME, AN IN-DEPTH LOOK

Reading this chapter is optional. If you have an interest in anatomy and like to get an in-depth understanding of things, this chapter is for you. If you would rather just stick with the basics, feel free to skip this one.

Hiatal hernia encompasses an incredibly long list of symptoms.

In order for a clinician to treat it successfully, they need to possess not only a full understanding of its anatomy, but they further must possess a root cause mindset, which allows them to comprehensively evaluate the hiatal hernia sufferer from a lens that includes structural, neurological, dietary, hormonal and digestive systems.

Few doctors are trained to think this way, which is likely why you have continued to suffer. It is a problem we hope this book helps in some way to improve.

In this chapter we are going to review the diaphragm, its anatomy, and how it interrelates with many muscles, major nerves, and organs in your body.

This chapter explains why there is the need to evaluate a number of areas of your body if you want to successfully treat Hiatal Hernia Syndrome.

Structurally, your neck, middle back, lower back, hips, and abdomen – along with muscles, nerves and tendons – must all be evaluated.

This anatomical review will also help explain why the successful treatment of Hiatal Hernia Syndrome is not a single step or a single procedure.

Success in treatment is very much dependent upon the proper analysis of what is imbalanced or malfunctioning within each individual. It is a personalized treatment program.

The Diaphragm

The diaphragm consists of two dome-shaped muscles separating your chest from your abdominal organs.

The diaphragm is your major muscle of inspiration (drawing air into your lungs). As you inhale, the diaphragm pulls down your lower ribs, creating a vacuum-like effect that "sucks" air into your lungs. The diaphragm has some non-respiratory functions as well. While it draws air in, it simultaneously pushes the abdominal organs down, creating abdominal pressure that helps rid your body of waste products, feces and urine.

When you exhale, air is pushed out, and now there is a negative pressure on the abdominal organs. Therefore, your diaphragm is much more than a vehicle for air exchange. Through the vacuum effect, it also helps with circulation and excretion within your digestive tract.

Your diaphragm is "anchored" to your spine by two tendons. These tendinous structures are called crura (singular is crus). Crus means "leg" in Latin. They take their name from their "leg-shaped" appearance.

The crus extend below the diaphragm to the spine on each side. Together they act as a tether for muscular contraction.

The next step of inspiration, once the downward movement of the abdominal organs has reached its limit, is that the diaphragm elevates first the lower ribs and then the upper ribs to expand the size of the thoracic cage.

Thus, there is a balance of abdominal downward movement and thoracic (or chest) outward movement, allowing for the full depth of respiration.

The design of the muscles of the diaphragm surrounding the opening of the esophagus is fascinating. The tendons (crura) of the diaphragm surround the opening and provide a scissors-like or pinching action on the esophagus to aid in maintaining the competence of the esophageal sphincter.

The crura (tendons) are exerting a supplementary, or back-up, "sphincter-like" action on the lower end of the esophagus. By design they relax after you swallow, allowing the contents moving down the esophagus to enter your stomach, only to immediately contract again after the bolus of food has passed into your stomach.

Too often attention is only given to the sphincter of the esophagus, forgetting about the additional "sphincter-like" action performed by your diaphragm.

Diaphragm attachments

Breathing adequately and easily is obviously critical to sustain life. It should not come as a surprise that your diaphragm anchors itself in a variety of areas in your body, to ensure you get enough oxygen.

Below is the list of diaphragm attachments:

- Xiphoid process (the tip of your sternum)
- Ribs, the lower six
- Esophageal opening, the left side
- Transverse abdominal muscle (the muscle layer beneath your oblique abdominal muscles, which layers across the front and side of your abdominal wall)
- Fronts and sides of the lumbar spine vertebrae (the bones of your lower back)
- Psoas (pronounced SO-az) muscle. You have two psoas muscles, one on each side. They are the deepest muscles in your core, originating from the lower spine vertebrae and the bottom of your rib cage (psoas minor), running down through your pelvis to the inner side of your femur, or thigh bone. The muscles flex your hip joint and lift your thigh towards your body. They are the only muscles that connect your spine to your legs. If you spend a lot of

time sitting (and who does not?) your psoas can become tight; the chronic sitting shortens it. Walking also uses this muscle. The psoas is a postural muscle, stabilizing your spine. It is the major connector between your torso and legs.

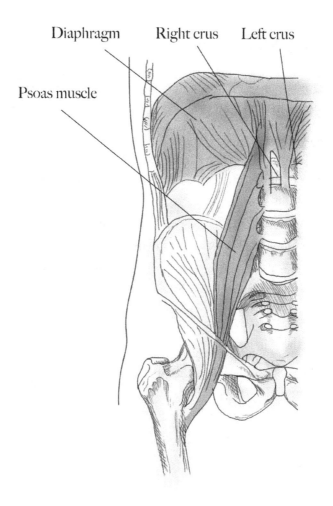

Diaphragm   Right crus   Left crus

Psoas muscle

- Quadratus lumborum muscle. This is your deepest abdominal muscle. It is a common cause of low back pain when it is in spasm. It originates from your lowest rib and ends at the top of your pelvis, contributing to the stabilization and movement of your lower back and pelvis. This muscle is used when sitting, standing, and walking.

Openings in the diaphragm

There are large and small openings in your diaphragm through which a variety of organ structures, nerves and blood vessels pass.

Three large openings for:

- Esophagus (the tube connecting your mouth to your stomach)
- Aorta (a large artery, your largest, carrying oxygenated blood to all parts of your body)
- Vena cava (a large vein, again your largest, carrying deoxygenated blood back to the heart from all parts of your body).

There are also several smaller openings: one is at the level of the lower middle back where the phrenic nerve (described below) passes through.

Nerves

Nerves need to function properly in order to send proper signals to the muscles they innervate, or control, as well as to communicate to your brain what action is being performed.

The diaphragm is a muscle, but we also just listed a number of muscles your diaphragm attaches to. All must be functioning properly for your diaphragm to move as it should.

Nerves traveling to your diaphragm

Your brain communicates to your diaphragm through the phrenic nerves, which exit from both sides of the middle of your neck. Specifically, the third, fourth and fifth cervical (neck) vertebrae.

This is where a chiropractic adjustment of the neck can be very impactful in diaphragmatic function. Normalizing the nerve flow from the brain to your diaphragm can be effected at the level of your neck.

The quadratum lumborum muscle (QL) attaches to your twelfth (last) rib, and it must be operating properly so the diaphragm can provide the maximum downward thrust on the abdominal organs during the latter half of inspiration. The nerves traveling to the quadratum lumborum muscle must also function correctly in order for the muscle to function properly. These nerves come from your lower back.

The psoas muscle is frequently reactive with the diaphragm and is a common cause of diaphragmatic dysfunction. The nerves that control the psoas muscle originate from your upper lumbar (lower back) vertebrae, levels one through three.

There is a technique called a psoas release which is performed by our Doctor of Physical Therapy that can impact the normalization of diaphragm function tremendously. Few would appreciate the importance of evaluating this muscle's function as it relates to Hiatal Hernia Syndrome. We find it, however, to be a common problem.

Hopefully, this chapter has provided some depth of understanding of the complexity of your diaphragm and all the structures that can influence it. It hopefully also explains why efficacious treatment includes physical treatment, physical therapy and chiropractic, and not just internal treatment of the diet and digestive tract.

CHAPTER 7

WHAT PUTS YOU AT RISK OF HIATAL HERNIA SYNDROME?

As the incidence of hiatal hernia continues to rise in our practice, we have isolated risk factors that are common amongst those who suffer.

Hiatal hernia occurs in both sexes and all ages. We see the condition in young men and women in their twenties.

The risk does tend to increase with age, with the predominant age group being individuals from forty to seventy years old. It is estimated that up to sixty percent of individuals age sixty suffer with Hiatal Hernia Syndrome.

Due to the increased risk of cardiovascular disease in this age group, the symptoms common in HHS can also indicate a heart attack or other coronary event.

Symptoms common in HHS include heart palpitations; chest pain;

49

shortness of breath; pain that can radiate into the neck, left arm, chest, back and jaw. But those same symptoms are common in an individual having a heart attack.

Therefore, it is important to get your heart checked out as a priority if these symptoms are present. Once it is confirmed there is nothing wrong with your heart, then we can get to the real root of your symptoms.

Common risk factors

Inflammation

Inflammation is the root of all degenerative diseases and is a response by your immune system. Eighty percent of the human immune system is housed in your gut, so a problem with inflammation will be a stressor on gut health and vice versa. Diseases associated with inflammation are many, including the leading killers such as heart disease, diabetes, cancer, autoimmune disease, and obesity.

Our "SAD" American diet

SAD is an abbreviation for Standard American Diet, and it is (sadly) a very poor one. Diets that are sugar-laden, highly processed, rich in chemicals, preservatives, bad fats, and (in the case of animal products) hormone-laden are not a formula for health.

It is estimated that sixty percent of what all Americans eat is ultra-processed "food" that should not even be called food. It is high in calories, nutritionally deficient and is the cause of inflammation.

Such a diet puts a great strain on your digestive tract, causing bloating, gas, constipation, and weight gain, which can contribute to Hiatal Hernia Syndrome.

Magnesium deficiency

Magnesium is required for the functioning of over three hundred enzymes in the body, with ninety percent of magnesium found in your bones and muscles.

Fifty percent of Americans consume inadequate magnesium for their bodies' needs.

Magnesium will reduce spasming of the esophageal sphincter, preventing the release of acid up into the esophagus. Considering the prevalence of magnesium deficiency, it would be prudent to evaluate this as one potential causative factor of your hiatal hernia or GERD.

Magnesium is also required for the stomach to produce adequate stomach acid. While it sounds counter-intuitive, symptoms of heartburn can be due to insufficient stomach acid.

Hypertension, high blood pressure, and heart arrhythmias are additional symptoms of magnesium deficiency.

Lack of exercise

Exercise tends to induce heavy breathing as you require more oxygen to get through whatever exercise you are performing.

Exercise is not only good for your circulation, brain, and the integrity of your muscles, it's also a good workout for a muscle related to Hiatal Hernia Syndrome: your diaphragm.

Regular exercise keeps your diaphragm strong and in motion due to deep breathing. Using your diaphragm often and getting it to move to its capacity helps "massage" the stomach into place.

Shallow breathing, or chest breathing, is not healthy for your diaphragm.

Stress

Stress is not good for anything when it is chronic, so it should not come as a surprise that it is a negative when it comes to Hiatal Hernia Syndrome as well.

Have you ever been under stress and felt "butterflies in your stomach"? Or perhaps the stress was more intense, and you found yourself running to the bathroom with diarrhea? If you have had such experiences, you know the connection between stress and your digestive tract.

The gut, like most organs of your body, is controlled (at least partly) by the central nervous system in the brain and spinal cord. Your digestive tract has a network of neurons (nerves) in the lining of your gut called the enteric or intrinsic nervous system.

This system of nerves is so powerful that many researchers have come to consider the gut as a second brain. The enteric nervous system has one hundred million nerve cells lining your gut from top (your esophagus) to bottom (your rectum.)

These nerves regulate swallowing, the release of enzymes to digest food, the absorption of nutrients, plus the elimination of waste products.

One aspect of your nervous system is the autonomic nervous system. It is often referred to as the "automatic" part of your nervous system since it is responsible for systems that are largely unconscious. As an example, you do not have to tell your heart to beat – it happens automatically. The same is true for breathing, digestion, etc.

The counterpart to your autonomic nervous system is your somatic nervous system. This is involved with voluntary actions you are aware of. An example of this is "deciding" to move your arm or leg or speak.

The autonomic (automatic) nervous system has two parts: sympathetic and parasympathetic. You are likely familiar with the sympathetic nervous system, which is often referred to as the "fight or flight" part of your nervous system.

Stress activates your fight or flight nervous system. With fight or flight, you get a surge of adrenaline, more blood is pumped to your muscles, your memory is more acute, and you get more oxygen flowing. Fight or flight is designed to make you extra strong to fight an opponent, or extra fast to flee a dangerous scene.

Proper digestion, on the other hand, requires activation of the parasympathetic system, also known as the rest, digest, repair, regenerate part of your nervous system.

What is important to know is that you cannot digest effectively if you are under stress. The activities of fight or flight are in direct opposition to digesting, relaxing and, of note, having your immune system work properly.

"Good" stress and being in fight or flight is fine as long as it's temporary. You are excited about something, you have a presentation at work, or even a fun activity with friends. Exercise will put you into fight or flight. It is great; but it is designed to be temporary.

Proper and effective digestion does not occur in the presence of stress – just the opposite, in fact.

The sympathetic nervous system accomplishes successful fight or flight by regulating your heart rate, breathing and blood pressure. It releases the stress hormone cortisol to put you on high alert, ready to successfully face the threat, whatever it may be.

This stress response is brilliant, truly a life saver when it is deployed appropriately. You breathe faster and pump more blood to your heart and muscles, becoming faster, stronger, and more alert and aware, to better face the stressful situation.

When faced with a true stressful situation, your body will not be engaged in digestion. It directs its efforts toward motion and strength, the very opposite of what needs to occur in healthy digestion.

However, if you are eating and trying to digest your food, and a stress response occurs inappropriately, it will really compromise your digestion.

If you've ever gobbled down a meal quickly because you were in a rush and stressed, only to have it sit in your stomach like "a rock," then you've experienced the bad blend of trying to digest while in fight or flight mode.

When stress activates your sympathetic (fight or flight) nervous system, you may experience the following:

- A spasm in your esophagus. Have you ever eaten in a "rush" and gotten something "stuck" in your throat? That is what we are describing.

- Increased stomach acid. Have you been under stress and gotten a stomach upset or a "sour stomach"? This is an example.

- Nausea. Perhaps you have had the experience of eating under stress, then feeling so nauseous you wish you had skipped the meal.

- Diarrhea or constipation. Two extremes for sure, but both are indicative of imbalanced digestive processes. In the case of diarrhea, the body is so stressed that it just wants to get rid of what you ate quickly, not taking the time to efficiently digest. With constipation, the stress has slowed the process (the other extreme), and you are unable to pass the toxins from your body in a timely manner.

- If stress is more extreme, you may feel cramping, extreme pain. "My gut is in a knot" is an expression that describes this well. The lack of blood flow to the digestive tract is causing inflammation, cramping and an imbalance of healthy gut microbes.

This situation can exacerbate such conditions as GERD, peptic ulcers, IBS (irritable bowel syndrome), and IBD (irritable bowel disease).

It's a lot easier said than done to "control your stress levels," but it may be of value to you to understand this association so that you can take whatever measures possible to not eat while you are feeling especially stressed.

Unfortunately, when you are stressed your body produces stress hormones that steer you in unhealthy directions.

Have you heard of "mindful eating"? Well, its opposite is "mindless eating" and unfortunately that is what you tend to do when really stressed out. Have you ever eaten a whole bag of chips, a whole pint of ice cream, or a large bag of candy without quite realizing it? That is classic mindless eating. It not only involves overeating – a big no-no for hiatal hernia – but you tend to crave the foods that have the worst effect on your health. Unfortunately, it is the high-salt, high-sugar, high-bad-fat foods that always sound the best when you are under stress.

Some stress reducing foods

- Salmon, which is rich in omega-3 fatty acids that can boost your mood and are beautifully anti-inflammatory.

- Magnesium (mentioned earlier) is a nice relaxer to your system, proven to calm cortisol levels. Avocados are rich in magnesium, as are almonds.

- Legumes (including lentils, beans, chickpeas, peas, and soybeans) are nutrient-dense foods that are also full of healthy, relaxing magnesium.

- Finally, seeds such as flax, pumpkin and chia are another great source of this mineral.

Please visit CHAPTER 15: RECIPES for healthy menu suggestions.

You also tend to eat quickly when you are under stress, another big contraindication for Hiatal Hernia Syndrome.

When you are under stress you tend to hold your breath and/or breathe shallowly. As mentioned above under lack of exercise, this failure to give your diaphragm a good workout prevents the diaphragm from "massaging" your stomach, along with other upper abdominal organs - functions important to maintaining their correct position.

Obesity or overweight

Over seventy percent of Americans are overweight, and over forty percent are obese. Sadly, every time we assess this figure rises. Carrying around excess weight in your midsection increases intra-abdominal pressure and weakens the muscles of your core, all potential contributors to Hiatal Hernia Syndrome.

Weight reduction is important, especially belly weight. Losing just ten pounds can make a big difference in the stress on your diaphragm. If you have a lot of weight to lose, don't despair. Little changes will yield big results if you keep them up.

It's also important to avoid straining the diaphragm with actions such as bending over, eating excessively large meals, lifting heavy weights, or straining during bowel movements.

Pregnancy

Certainly, a legitimate reason for increased belly weight, but sometimes mom can gain an excessive amount of weight and it can put extra pressure on the digestive organs, especially the stomach.

Women who gain a tremendous amount of weight during pregnancy put themselves at extra risk. Instead of twenty to twenty-five pounds, some gain fifty to eighty pounds. This excess weight puts a burden on your gut.

Sometimes babies can be large or just not in the "right" place. There is nothing like a well-placed baby foot to give mommy acid reflux. This latter situation is typically alleviated with the birth of the child. (From Dr. Vikki: I well remember being pregnant with my first – a large baby – and experiencing my very first occurrence of acid reflux. I was instantly sympathetic to my patients who suffered with it chronically.)

Diastasis recti

While we are discussing pregnancy, let's look at a common side effect where the normal spreading of the abdominal muscles does not mend correctly after pregnancy.

A diastasis is the thinning and weakening of the linea alba, a vertical line of connective tissue connecting the left and right sides of your abdominal muscles (rectus abdominus). Think of "six-pack abs": the vertical line running down the middle is the linea alba.

It most commonly occurs during pregnancy but can also be the result of weight gain in the abdomen.

As many as sixty-six percent of women in their final trimester of pregnancy experience it, and many do not heal on their own after the birth of baby, as they should. It is estimated that thirty to sixty percent of women post-partum (after pregnancy) continue to suffer with the condition.

Those at risk are moms who have delivered a high birth-weight baby, have a multiple pregnancy (e.g. twins), or women who deliver babies when they are over the age of thirty-five.

Men are not off the hook: middle-aged and older men with extra belly weight are also at risk.

Many women, post pregnancy, call diastasis recti their "pooch." It is a noticeable bulge in the middle of the abdomen. It can also be less noticeable, only appearing with tensing of the abdominal muscles, such as during a cough or when bearing down.

Here at Root Cause Medical Clinic our Doctor of Physical Therapy performs the treatment that can rebuild the thickness of the linea alba, strengthen the deeper abdominal muscles, and "re-condition" the rectus abdominus.

In rare (extreme) cases surgery is required to regain the integrity of the abdominal muscles.

While hiatal hernia does not cause diastasis recti, diastasis recti can be a stressor (due to the weakness of the abdominal musculature) that can increase your risk of Hiatal Hernia Syndrome.

Abdominal hernias

Abdominal hernias are quite common and are among the most frequently performed surgeries in the U.S., where up to 500,000 abdominal hernia surgeries are performed each year. Most of these patients (three to one ratio) are men.

Abdominal hernias and hiatal hernias share many associated risk factors, such as chronic constipation, obesity, chronic cough, and lifting heavy weight.

Constipation

Acute or chronic constipation is extremely common in our Hiatal Hernia Syndrome patients.

From a physical standpoint, constipation tends to involve straining or bearing down to pass stool. Bearing down increases intra-abdominal pressure which can cause an upward push upon the diaphragm and stomach.

We are not talking about a one-time experience, or constipation that occurs rarely. The person with the common risk factor for hiatal hernia is currently suffering or has suffered chronically in the past.

Defining constipation is important because we frequently meet patients who move their bowels every other day or less, but who do not consider it a problem. If you have never moved your bowels daily, you would not find it unusual, but a true "normal" frequency is once or twice a day. The stool should be easy to pass, require no straining nor bearing down, and resemble a "brown banana" in length and diameter. It is formed and should stay formed in the toilet. The stool's color should be brown, not black, tan nor yellow.

We understand that your doctor may have told you that "it's fine" or "it's normal for you" but we disagree. We have been treating patients for decades, and once their digestive tract is normalized, everyone moves their bowels daily.

The presence of stool that has been residing in the intestine for too long creates a host of problems. Bad bacteria proliferate, and when you do try to move your bowels, any straining or bearing down increases the intra-abdominal pressure within your gut, an absolute risk factor for Hiatal Hernia Syndrome.

Coughing

Chronic or strong coughing can initiate a hiatal hernia. If you have had an infection that has left you with a strong or lingering cough, the strong intra-abdominal pressure created from a chronic cough can push your diaphragm and stomach upwards.

Vomiting

This too creates a strong intra-abdominal pressure that can force your stomach upwards.

One episode of vomiting should not cause a problem, but if you are vomiting often, for whatever reason, this can put you at risk of hiatal hernia.

Lifting heavy objects

This is a lifestyle factor that we often see in our younger patients with hiatal hernia. Whether you're a weight-lifter that pushes some heavy weights or someone who is required to lift heavy objects at work, the strain of lifting improperly, or beyond the capability of your abdominal and core muscles, can put you at risk of hiatal hernia.

Improper lifting is a common mechanical cause of hiatal hernia. Do you remember the adage "lift with your legs, not with your back?" How about this one: "Inhale as you relax into the starting position of any exercise, and exhale on the lifting part, or the tough part."

You want to take a nice deep belly breath (the type of breath that utilizes your diaphragm) just before you lift a heavy weight. Using your diaphragm allows you to get a nice, deep full breath that fills your lungs with the oxygen needed for exercise. It also helps to stabilize the muscles of your abdomen, back, and sides – all your core muscles. It also stabilizes your spine.

With your lungs full of air in preparation, you will naturally exhale as you lift the weight.

> **Note:** if you do not feel able to get a deep breath, or tend to feel light-headed when exercising, this could indicate the presence of Hiatal Hernia Syndrome.

A good question to address is: What is too heavy? This varies depending on the strength of the individual.

You may have always lifted heavy objects at work, but now you are older, have gained twenty pounds, or your abdominal muscles are weaker. The poundage is the exact same, but you are less able to successfully deal with it.

Body builders and those lifting very heavy weight may be extremely strong and in amazing shape but decide to "up" their weight just beyond their tolerable threshold. The result is strain and an increase of intra-abdominal pressure to the point of forcing the diaphragm and stomach upwards.

Sit-ups

Exercise is very healthy, and correctly performed sit-ups with nice exhalation during the sitting up motion are incredibly important to retain core strength. Sit-ups, however, are not your friend while you are suffering from an active hiatal hernia. Once your condition is resolved you can build back up to sit-ups, but that should be under the advice of a savvy physical therapist or Doctor of Chiropractic, well-versed in the problem.

Sit-ups increase the intra-abdominal pressure in much the same way as lifting excessive weight can.

Lower back pain or weakness of the psoas muscle

When someone comes in with Hiatal Hernia Syndrome and major digestive complaints, they understandably find it odd when we ask if they have any lower back issues or posture complaints.

A little anatomy will clear up the strong association between the two conditions. CHAPTER 6 of this book does a deep dive into anatomy. If you chose to skip it, let me give you a quick overview.

The psoas (SO-az) muscle lies deep in your core, originating from the lower spine vertebrae and the bottom of your rib cage (psoas minor), running down through your pelvis to the inner side of your femur, or thigh bone.

Your diaphragm, the main muscle of breathing, pulls downward to expand your chest cavity and inflate your lungs.

Your psoas, the main muscle of walking, is intimately connected to your diaphragm; they come together at your solar plexus. Literally with every breath you take, and with every step you take, these two muscles work together.

They provide stability to the front part of your spine and if you have poor posture, neither of them will work correctly.

The psoas muscle goes beyond just a structural component of your body: large bundles of nerves affecting your enteric (gut) nervous system, along with your sympathetic and central nervous system, all pass through the muscle.

The psoas affects your internal organs due to its positioning. It acts as a shelf to support your digestive organs in concert with your pelvis and pelvic floor. Thus, its contraction stimulates a variety of organs including your stomach, liver, pancreas, intestines, kidney, spleen, and bladder.

If the psoas is tight, which is quite common, it does not just affect you structurally: it can constrict organs, interfere with the circulation of fluids in your organs, put pressure on nerves and, as mentioned earlier, impair your diaphragmatic breathing.

There are some references mentioning that a tight psoas muscle can affect the position of the diaphragm around the stomach such that it can lead to trapped acid in the upper stomach.

A tight psoas muscle will cause symptoms of bloating, constipation, poor posture, chronic back pain, and even emotional stress due to its effect on your sympathetic (fight or flight) nervous system.

Isn't it incredible how a muscle of your lower back has the ability to affect so many parts of your body? We think so.

Tight clothing

This is a less significant contributor, and if you have been suffering for a while with Hiatal Hernia Syndrome you have likely intuitively figured this out. Along with other contributing factors that are preventing the easy movement of your diaphragm and creating a spasm of your stomach or esophagus, tight-fitting clothing can most definitely exacerbate the symptoms of Hiatal Hernia Syndrome.

History of neck pain, whiplash, or injury to the neck

You have learned how your lower back can be related to hiatal hernia. In much the same way the neck, which seems a long way from your stomach, can also be a causative factor.

You have seven bones (vertebrae) in your neck. The middle ones (numbers three, four, and five) provide the channel for the nerve that travels to your diaphragm from your brain. The same area has nerves controlling your face, teeth and lungs.

When any of those vertebrae are misaligned (called a subluxation), the nerve branch going to your diaphragm – called the phrenic (fren-ick) nerve – can be compromised in its function.

The phrenic nerve provides the diaphragm with the "nerve transmission" it needs to move properly and give you the ability to breathe freely and deeply.

If the nerve is functioning improperly, it can cause symptoms such as shortness of breath, anxiety, hiccupping, vertigo, and fatigue. As you can see, these are common symptoms associated with Hiatal Hernia Syndrome.

This is where chiropractic care can come in as a part of your treatment for Hiatal Hernia Syndrome.

Since this same phrenic nerve travels to your face and teeth, we will also ensure you have no other symptoms associated with its malfunction, such as:

- Jaw tightness
- Jaw pain, clenching your teeth
- Grinding your teeth
- Headaches

All the above are potential indicators of phrenic nerve malfunction.

Muscle weakness associated with aging

There is nothing you can do to stop the clock, it is true, but you do not have to get older and weaker at the same time. With advancing age can come a lack of exercise and weight gain, all resulting in weaker abdominal muscles and a generalized weakness of the entire abdomen and core. The body is an amazing machine: it loves to heal and get stronger.

Surgery of the abdomen

It only makes sense that abdominal surgery can result in a host of issues regarding the natural and normal integrity of your abdomen. Certainly, cutting into the abdomen will create some weakness in your muscles, hopefully temporary. Depending on the type of surgery, abdominal organs can literally get moved around. Once you have healed enough to be ambulatory, it is smart to address any weakness or loss of integrity that you may experience with an experienced clinician.

Genetics

It is uncommon, hence left for last on the list, but some individuals are born with an opening in their diaphragm that is larger than normal, putting them at greater risk for developing hiatal hernia.

Many of the risk factors we have just discussed are interrelated. To give you an example: a patient who is chronically constipated typically suffers from some form of inflammation, potentially has a poor diet, and may also be overweight and exercise infrequently.

That patient has a variety of compounding conditions, all working against him and potentially resulting in Hiatal Hernia Syndrome.

CHAPTER 8

THE DOS AND DON'TS OF HIATAL HERNIA SYNDROME

My ultimate goal is to fully remedy why you developed Hiatal Hernia Syndrome (HHS) and fix it. While you are undergoing diagnosis and treatment with a practitioner who fully understands all the ramifications of the syndrome, it is good to know some basic tips that can make the journey easier for yourself.

The last thing you want to do is unwittingly aggravate your condition because you were unaware that it was adding stress to the condition.

The Don'ts

Diet is a big contributor and ultimately a major cause of Hiatal Hernia Syndrome. We will talk more about food sensitivities in the treatment chapter, but some foods that can inflame your stomach or esophagus, making acid reflux or GERD worsen, are the following:

Caffeine

There are varying reactions when it comes to caffeine. For some, the caffeine relaxes the sphincter of the esophagus, worsening your reflux. Other patients find that one cup of coffee after eating some food is fine, but the same cup on an empty stomach creates problems.

Try coffee with or without food and see if there is a happy medium for you or if, for now, caffeine is simply too irritating.

Simple coffee or tea might be fine but avoid energy drinks: along with high amounts of caffeine, these are also full of other unhealthy ingredients. The same goes for caffeinated sodas. Sodas should not be in anyone's diet.

Carbonated beverages

Carbonation can increase pressure in your stomach, placing it at risk of reflux. The added pressure not only aggravates acid reflux, but can also cause burping, chest pain or shortness of breath. Even a carbonated water with no unhealthy ingredients can aggravate your condition, simply due to the carbonation alone. It is prudent to mention that sodas are full of sugar, high fructose corn syrup, and artificial ingredients, and should be avoided due to the unhealthy profile they present.

Artificial sweeteners

Avoid all artificial sweeteners. We do not include stevia or monk fruit on this list; although they have zero calories, they are made from plants and therefore not artificial.

Artificial sweeteners are troublesome for the gut microbiome, eliminating a good percentage of your gut's good bacteria. They are also inflammatory to your nervous system. They are never a good idea, but if you are suffering from heart palpitations, anxiety, or panic attacks due to your hiatal hernia, the last thing you need is another ingredient to stress your nervous system.

Fried, greasy or fatty foods

You have likely had the experience of eating an abundance of fat, then feeling heavy or lethargic. Fat can be more burdensome to digest when eaten in excess, and when your digestive tract is not functioning optimally, even a moderate amount of fat can be troublesome.

One of the problems so common with digestive problems is poor bile flow from the liver. Bile emulsifies or digests fats, but it also acts as a detergent for the upper intestine, keeping it clean of inhospitable organisms.

Our poor-quality American diets, along with increasing toxicity levels, often put a strain on our liver and its bile flow is compromised. The result is trouble digesting fats, making you feel bloated and full easily.

Spicy and acidic foods

Citrus, onions, and tomatoes (including tomato sauce and catsup) may relax the sphincter of your esophagus, aggravating your reflux. When it comes to other spicy foods, including peppers, they can aggravate your condition, but are typically not the cause of it.

Here is an example: imagine you have a small paper cut. It is quite small, and you have not noticed it while going about your day. You then pick up a lemon wedge to squeeze into your water – now you know you have the cut!

Think about this: did the lemon cause the paper cut or simply find the cut that was already there? It is the latter. You had the cut and the acidic lemon let you know the cut was present.

We find this is the same condition with spicy and acidic foods. You may not be able to tolerate onions or tomatoes or jalapeno peppers because your stomach or esophagus is inflamed. Once that inflammation is addressed however, you should typically be able to tolerate such foods again.

Garlic and onions

Along with their allium family "relatives" – shallot, leeks, chives and green onions – garlic and onions are in a "maybe" category when it comes to heartburn-inducing foods.

The allium family of foods can impart great health benefits, including protection from cardiovascular disease. They have blood pressure-, cholesterol- and triglyceride-lowering abilities, plus anti-cancer activity. Garlic and onions may be pungent, but they are highly anti-inflammatory.

Some blame the fermentable fiber in onions as it can cause belching, thereby aggravating acid reflux symptoms. Raw onions are highly acidic, but you can try cooking them (and garlic) to see if you can tolerate them.

It is well worth it to test these healthy foods so you are not eliminating them unnecessarily.

Peppermint and other types of mint

Mint can sound soothing, especially a nice cup of mint tea, but it can increase acid production in your stomach, creating a trigger for heartburn.

All refined vegetable oils

These include canola oil, corn oil, soybean oil, anything labeled "vegetable oil", safflower oil, sunflower oil, grapeseed oil, peanut oil, cottonseed oil, margarine, shortening or any fake butters.

This is a long list, we know, but it is important for your general health to avoid these oils at all costs, even once your Hiatal Hernia Syndrome is resolved.

Vegetable oils are extracted from various seeds and plants, but unlike the straightforward process that creates olive, avocado and coconut oil, the process used for these oils is complex and far from natural.

Let us take canola oil as an example. There is no canola seed nor canola plant. Canola oil is extracted from the rapeseed plant, a genetically modified plant that is typically treated with heavy pesticides.

The rapeseeds are heated to a high temperature, causing oxidation and rancidity (meaning the oil is "spoiled"). In order to extract the oil, it is processed with a petroleum solvent. It then goes through more heating and chemical treatment and finally is "deodorized" because all the chemical treatments leave a terrible smell. Scary, isn't it?

Getting a balance of oils in your diet is important, but your emphasis should be on those high in omega-3 fatty acids because they are anti-inflammatory, anti-cancer and protective of your brain and nervous system. In the American diet, omega-6 fatty acids are readily available; in fact, they are too readily available. You therefore do not need to worry about getting enough omega-6s, but rather the opposite. The omega-6 fatty acids are pro-inflammatory and Hiatal Hernia Syndrome has inflammation as an underlying factor.

The balance of omega-3s and 6s is really key, and despite the fact that omega-6s are pro-inflammatory, you do require some degree of inflammation for your immune system to fight foreign invaders such as bacteria, viruses and the like. The ratio between the two ideally should be about three to one, with the omega-6s as the higher amount.

The average American, sadly, has a ratio closer to sixteen or even twenty-two to one i.e. extremely out of balance and highly pro-inflammatory.

You can see why we advise you to focus more on getting omega-3s.

This dietary advice is good generally, even once your Hiatal Hernia Syndrome is fully under control. Americans should focus on consuming the fats highest in omega-3 fatty acids, which does not include the above-mentioned vegetable oils.

Over and above the amount of omega-6 fatty acids, the vegetable oils are unstable and therefore oxidize, or go rancid, easily. They are little "time bombs" of bad fats that you truly need to avoid. Of course, the manufacturers of these oils are very aware of their instability and attempt to handle this weakness with the addition of additives and chemicals, all added during processing. These chemicals do help with spoilage, but they are dangerous and have been associated with cancer, liver and kidney damage, hormonal imbalance, and immune system weakness.

This list of bad oils likely prompts the question: What are the good oils?

Here is a quick overview. Even within these good oils, organic and cold-pressed should be on the label. Basically, you are looking for an oil that has been minimally processed and is not heavy in omega-6 fatty acids.

- Avocado oil. This is made very simply by pressing avocado pulp – cold-pressed is best. It is high in monosaturated fat, considered to be the best when it comes to oils. It can be safely heated to high temperatures when cooking without destroying its integrity. Avocado oil has a very mild taste that will not impart any flavor to what you are cooking. Try to get organic.

- Extra-virgin olive oil. Similar to avocado oil, it's simply made from the pressing of whole olives. Organic is best, as is cold-pressed. The extra-virgin refers to the very first press of the olive, which is purest. Again, olive oil is highest in monounsaturated fats, making it the healthiest of oils. The caveat with olive oil is that it cannot sustain high heat without becoming altered. Therefore, cook with it only on very low heat. Even better, enjoy your olive oil in dressings or drizzle it over foods that have already been cooked.

- Coconut oil. A saturated fat, coconut oil should be used only in moderation and only for those individuals who do not suffer from elevated cholesterol. Like the two oils above, the process to make it is simple: just a pressing of the coconut meat is all that is required. Organic and cold expeller-pressed are best. It is said that expeller-pressed lessens the coconut flavor, if that is something you are trying to avoid in the dish you are preparing. Coconut oil is very high-heat stable.

Highly processed foods high in synthetic additives and chemicals

This most definitely includes fast food restaurants. American grocery shelves are teeming with "food" that should not be called food. It is so highly processed and contains so many chemical ingredients that it should be called a chemical additive rather than a food product. Deli meats are on this list.

These "foods" are so heavily laden with preservatives and chemicals they do not spoil. Real food should rot. There is a picture we use of a McDonald's "happy meal" when we lecture. The happy meal looks the same 180 days (six months) after it is prepared. Yet a slice of watermelon looks like a "green steak" a mere sixty days (two months) after it is cut. If a "food" has a long shelf life, and its ingredient list is long and sounds like a chemistry experiment, best to avoid it.

Again, this advice is true for everyone, not just for those suffering with Hiatal Hernia Syndrome. Such highly processed foods are inflammatory and will aggravate a hiatal hernia condition.

Chocolate and cocoa

If eating chocolate or cocoa-containing foods seems to bother your Hiatal Hernia Syndrome, you are not alone. It is a double-edged sword: cocoa can cause your body to make serotonin, that feel-good brain chemical that makes so many of us love and crave chocolate. Unfortunately, it is not so "feel good" for your esophageal sphincter. Serotonin can cause your sphincter to relax, allowing the acid and contents of your stomach to move upwards, aggravating your condition.

The caffeine in chocolate can also exacerbate your condition, due to its acidic nature and your already irritated esophagus.[1]

Alcohol and nicotine

Other substances known to relax the esophageal sphincter include alcohol and nicotine. Hopefully we don't need to say any more about the hazards of smoking, but here you go: smoking increases inflammation, thereby increasing acid production in some. It also compromises muscle reflexes, which are important in proper digestion.

Alcohol is a known initiator of acid reflux and heavy consumption is a definite risk factor. Alcohol can damage the mucosal lining of your stomach and esophagus. The latter is already inflamed due to acid reflux, so adding to the irritation is a poor strategy.

Alcohol is also a toxin of sorts and this adds a burden to your liver which it likely does not need. Too often with Hiatal Hernia

1   healthline.com article *"Can You Eat Chocolate If You Have Acid Reflux?"* Medically reviewed by Deborah Weatherspoon, Ph.D., R.N., CRNA — Written by Ashley Marcin

Syndrome the liver is already functioning at a deficit, so it does not need any more stress.

Some red wine in moderation can be healthful but if you find it irritating, you will need to abstain until your condition is corrected. Certainly, hard alcohol is never a good idea beyond special occasions, and you will likely find it quite irritating if you suffer reflux.

High fat foods

This includes dairy products such as cheese, cream and ice cream, as well as red meat, sausage, and fried chicken – the "rich" foods that are on so many American restaurants' menus as well as dinner tables. Rich, oily, greasy food can make you miserable if you have a hiatal hernia.

Fatty foods can be difficult to digest, made worse when you are taking an antacid which limits your ability to properly break down the food in your stomach.

Part of Hiatal Hernia Syndrome can involve liver toxicity or insufficient bile production. Bile is a fat emulsifier; any burden on the liver already present will only worsen with fatty food ingestion.

If you have had your hiatal hernia for a while, this information is likely all too real for you and you have begun to avoid fatty foods on your own.

Salty food

Some studies have shown that a diet high in sodium may cause acid reflux, leading to GERD. Yet healthy people do not demonstrate the association. Does there have to be a predisposition? Were the salty foods also high processed, unhealthy foods? Likely. More research needs to be done. Salt can bother some people, but we would not rule it out, as long as the food you're eating is healthy.

The Dos of Diet and Lifestyle

We think it is interesting that the foods recommended to prevent heartburn are also squarely in the "foods to enhance health" category.

High-fiber foods (fruits, vegetables, legumes)

High-fiber foods including fruits, vegetables and legumes are beneficial. A diet low in animal fat (including dairy products) is also recommended. Healthy fats from the plant kingdom are a definite yes, along with adequate water ingestion. For some who tolerate whole, unadulterated grains, oatmeal is an example of a heartburn-preventing food.

The high-fiber foods factually reduce stomach acid, and they are low in fat. They start assisting digestion at the top of your digestive tract – your stomach – and continue their good work all the way down to your colon, where they enhance your microbiome or good bacteria.

It is interesting how fresh organic vegetables are always a "do" regardless of what health condition we are discussing. When it comes to Hiatal Hernia Syndrome, they once again top the list. Enjoy your dark leafy greens, asparagus, squash, and cucumbers, to name just a few.

Note: If raw veggies are difficult for you to digest, do not abandon veggies altogether. Just cook them and you will still derive their health benefits. Once your condition is resolved, you will once again be able to tolerate raw veggies and salads.

Fruits are also on the "do" list, berries making the very top. Avoid citrus if it bothers you; its acidic content can be aggravating to many with acid reflux.

Fish

If you eat fish, the SMASH fish are the best as they provide good protein and good fat, are easy to digest, and do not tend to bio-accumulate mercury as so many fish do.

SMASH is an acronym for: sardines, mackerel, anchovies, salmon, herring.

Other than the salmon, all the fish on the list are quite small, making them extremely safe when it comes to mercury hazards. The salmon should be wild-caught and from Alaska or the Pacific. Avoid Atlantic salmon, which is unhealthy.

Ginger

The benefits of ginger have long been recognized. It is anti-inflammatory and you can use it in your cooking or to make a tea to assist not only your heartburn, but your general gut health.

Herbs

Licorice is an herb that is known for its soothing and healing properties. There are some licorice teas and supplements. (Please note we are NOT discussing licorice candy here.)

Chamomile is another herb known to soothe the digestive tract. You can try a pure tea of chamomile to see if it helps your symptoms.

Herbs such as parsley and fennel have long been known for their antacid and soothing effects on the digestive tract.

Water

It may sound obvious, but since most Americans are dehydrated, it seems clear that water's neutral pH and ability to flush toxins from the body is often overlooked. We have met many patients whose stomach was so inflamed that even water bothered them. Obviously, the water is not causing the problem, but is rather aggravating a highly inflamed system.

You may have heard it is important to drink eight glasses of purified water each day. This is true, but the timing of the water is also important. Drink your water separate from meals. It is fine to have a glass of water between meals, but not during them. Why? Drinking while you eat dilutes your digestive juices, inhibiting ideal digestion and absorption. Allow a window of about forty-five to sixty minutes on either side of your meals, in which you do not drink anything.

Additionally, only drink one glass of water per hour. Guzzling more than eight ounces of water in an hour prevents you from obtaining all its detoxification abilities.

Probiotic-rich and fermented foods

These contain acid-reducing bacteria that can be calming and balancing to an irritated intestine. We are not fans of any animal-based yogurts but there are many plant-based options you can enjoy along with kombucha, sauerkraut, miso, tempeh and natto.

Apple cider vinegar (ACV)

Apple cider vinegar has long been known for its effect of creating alkalinity in the body, thereby reducing symptoms such as heartburn and GERD.

It is a bit counterintuitive since apple cider vinegar is decidedly acidic on the tongue. Very true, but its effect upon your body internally is quite the opposite. ACV is quite good at quelling acidity and can be of temporary relief for heartburn and GERD.

It does not work for everyone and it's not a cure, but if you were to compare side effects of antacid medications versus ACV, the vinegar wins every time. There is no harm in trying the vinegar while you are (hopefully) finding a clinician who will get to the true underlying cause of your heartburn or GERD and get it fixed for good.

Remember, acid reflux is a sign of imbalance which, if left uncorrected, can lead to a host of digestive and chronic system-wide imbalances. Do not just stop at the band-aid; find the cure.

Apple Cider Vinegar Drink Recipe

1. Add 1 to 2 teaspoons of raw, unfiltered organic apple cider vinegar to a glass of warm filtered water.
2. Sip it slowly before you eat.

3. Repeat whenever you have heartburn or acidity.

Aloe vera

Decolorized and purified aloe vera juice appears to be safe and effective in reducing acid reflux symptoms.

An interesting study published in the *Journal of Traditional Chinese Medicine* in December 2015[2] compared the effects of aloe to those of traditional acid reflux medications, given morning and night (specifically Omeprazole or a Ranitidine/Pepcid tablet).

Seventy-nine participants were randomized to the aloe vera group or the antacid drug group and given their treatment first thing in the morning on an empty stomach and again thirty minutes before bed at night. The study lasted four weeks.

The frequencies of eight main symptoms of GERD were evaluated: heartburn, food regurgitation, flatulence, belching, dysphagia (trouble swallowing), nausea, vomiting and acid regurgitation.

Participants were assessed at weeks two and four of the trial. The group receiving the aloe vera syrup experienced a reduction in frequency of all eight symptoms at both weeks two and four, compared to the baseline level at which they began the study.

Important to note, there were no intolerable effects created from the aloe vera.

When compared to the group taking the drugs, the drug group had a more significant reduction of the frequency of all the assessed

2   National Library of Medicine, PubMed.gov "*Efficacy and safety of Aloe vera syrup for the treatment of gastroesophageal reflux disease: a pilot randomized positive-controlled trial*"

GERD symptoms. It is worth noting, however, that the group who was administered the drugs had two patients drop out due to adverse side effects. The aloe vera group had zero dropouts.

The trial led by Panahi et al, concluded that aloe vera may provide safe and effective treatment for reducing the symptoms of GERD.

A study published a year later (2016) in the *Journal of the American Medical Association* (JAMA) came to similar conclusions[3].

The study suggested that the cause of acid reflux may very well be more closely related to inflammation than to the chemical injury caused by stomach acid. Aloe is particularly beneficial at reducing inflammation; it also has antioxidant properties.

We don't disagree with their conclusion.

The concerns associated with acid reducing medication are many, yet too often we find patients have no idea they should be concerned.

Research has linked proton pumps inhibitors (PPIs), a type of acid reflux medication, to an increased risk of hip fracture, dementia, enteric (within your digestive tract) infection and overgrowth, heart attack, and overall increased risk of death from heart disease, kidney disease and cellular aging (premature aging)[4].

> (**Note:** if you are currently taking an antacid, please re-read the above paragraph. The side effects of antacids are very serious – frankly, they are potentially life-threatening.)

In addition to GERD, numerous studies have demonstrated aloe's

---

3   Dunbar KB, Agoston AT, Odze RD, et al. *Association of acute gastroesophageal reflux disease with esophageal histologic changes.* JAMA. 2016;315(19):2104-2112.

4   Reference: Brisebois MD, et al. Laryngoscope Investig Otolaryngol. 2018 Dec; 3(6): 457–462. *Proton pump inhibitors: Review of reported risks and controversies*]

positive effects upon H. pylori infection (a bacterial infection of the stomach), IBS, peptic ulcer, and ulcerative colitis[5].

Healthy Weight

Finding and maintaining a healthy weight can be a tall order for many Americans who are overweight or obese. The structural truth of carrying too many pounds, especially in the abdominal area, is that it puts extra stress and pressure on the valve separating the esophagus and stomach.

As a further source of aggravation, obesity is often associated with lower levels of stomach acid, which may sound good if you suffer from acid reflux, but quite the contrary is true. Stomach acid is needed for proper digestion and absorption of your nutrients.

As weight and BMI (body mass index) increases, so too do symptoms of GERD.

Women who have been pregnant and have temporarily suffered acid reflux towards the end of their pregnancy have experienced what added belly weight can do. Suddenly they are carrying a lot more weight in their abdomen, and they suffer with reflux because their esophageal sphincter cannot maintain its integrity.

Fortunately, this type of acid reflux is typically temporary, and resolves naturally once baby is born. But for other women – either due to gaining too much weight which they're then unable to lose, or to the lack of healing of their abdominal muscles (called diastasis

---

5   Reference: J Tradit Chin Med. 2015 Dec;35(6):632-6. *Efficacy and safety of Aloe vera syrup for the treatment of gastroesophageal reflux disease: a pilot randomized positive-controlled trial.* Panahi Y, et al.]

recti) – their pregnancy is the start of a chronic condition which they'll require assistance to resolve.

Elevating the head of your bed

If you've ever awoken in the middle of the night choking from acid reflux or having a panic attack from heart palpitations or the anxiety that can be associated with your nervous system being on high alert, you've likely gone online at 2:00 or 3:00 a.m. and discovered that elevating the head of your bed can help relieve your symptoms.

The common recommendation is to raise the head of your bed six to eight inches, or whatever relieves your reflux symptoms. It does help some people quite a bit, but of course it is just a temporary solution while we get to the true root of your problem. Elevation can mitigate symptoms, but it is not a cure.

Sleeping on a wedge is another recommendation. It's best if the wedge is placed beneath your mattress – if it is placed on top of your mattress it can interfere with restful sleep due to the feeling of slipping down the wedge or not being able to move around comfortably.

If it is workable for you to raise the head of your bed with blocks, that is likely your best bet.

Do not go to sleep on a full stomach

Another night-time tip is to ensure at least a three-hour window after dinner before heading to bed. Eat a small meal, remembering to eat slowly and chew well. Relax and remain upright for three hours before lying down.

A relaxing walk after dinner can also assist digestion, ensuring your food has left your stomach before going to bed. Try not to be completely stationary. Some movement in a relaxed fashion is a great way to enhance digestion.

Exercise

Exercise is a "do" for almost everyone. The benefits include overall health and help with motility of the digestive tract, which can be especially important if you suffer constipation. Exercise is also helpful with detoxification, lowers inflammation, helps maintain cognitive or brain health and creates endorphins that help you feel less stressed.

The downside of exercise is something that must be addressed with Hiatal Hernia Syndrome, as there are some forms that can aggravate the condition. This is not to say that all exercise should be avoided, only that you will need to find what works for you.

Heavy weights (weightlifting) are a bad idea. They increase intra-abdominal pressure and can often aggravate the elevation of your stomach above your diaphragm.

Sit-ups are often a definite "no" as they increase the intra-abdominal pressure in much the same way lifting weights does.

Walking often makes patients feel better, but too brisk a walk can irritate shortness of breath.

Exercising on a full stomach is never a good idea, but it can be particularly aggravating if you have acid reflux. The best time to exercise for fat burning is first thing in the morning on an empty stomach. If your blood sugar is stable enough to exercise without eating, that would be very safe. Of course, consult your doctor if you are not sure if this advice suits your health condition.

There is no absolute when it comes to exercise other than this:

1. It is important to move the body.
2. Move it in such a way that you feel better and not worse.

This is not forever, but you do not want to be aggravating your condition with the wrong types of activities.

Managing Stress

Stress is such a major part of this condition that talking about "managing it" can be stressful in itself. We fully understand. If you are suffering heart palpitations, panic attacks, are barely eating or sleeping, stress is really impacting your life.

If you've visited the emergency room on one or more occasions due to heart palpitations and/or panic attacks, you've likely already been assured that your heart is fine and you're "only" having a panic attack, or the cause of your palpitations is unknown, but it's not your heart.

Most patients, after one or more emergency visits, learn to somewhat "deal" with these symptoms. It is never easy to have your heart beating out of your chest or to struggle with the extreme anxiety that besets you out of the blue. It is downright scary, and we truly fully understand.

Once you have determined that neither your heart nor lungs are at risk, and your condition is a hiatal hernia, doing your best to manage your stress in whatever fashion works for you is worth the effort.

Your body is under terrific stress internally when suffering from

Hiatal Hernia Syndrome, and unfortunately, stress only increases inflammation. Anything you can do to manage your mental stress and lessen any lifestyle stress besetting you will help.

Meal size

Beyond the good and bad choices already mentioned, the size of your meals and the speed at which you consume them is also something to be mindful of.

If you have had your condition for a while, you have already figured out that eating slowly, and small quantities in any given sitting, is helpful. Your stomach is in spasm and therefore it does not take as much to get it filled.

Eating slowly and chewing your food well will allow for digestion to occur without burdening your stomach and allowing it to over-fill. Many patients lose a lot of weight with this condition. This may be a bit of a plus if you have weight to lose, but the bottom line is this dysfunction is NOT ultimately of benefit to you and is not health-promoting, despite any "perk" of weight loss.

You must also assess what you are eating and ensure you are maintaining a balanced diet of healthful carbohydrates (vegetables and some fruits), fats and protein.

Taking a slow walk after eating can also enhance digestion as the movement of your body and gravity will assist your stomach to not spasm as much. Remember this is a slow walk, not a jog nor run.

CHAPTER 9

WHY DOCTORS DON'T TREAT THE HIATAL HERNIAS THEY FIND

It can be very frustrating to finally receive the diagnosis of hiatal hernia only to be told by your doctor that it creates no symptoms other than acid reflux.

As we discussed earlier, there are close to twenty different symptoms caused by Hiatal Hernia Syndrome (HHS), symptoms that are incompatible with a healthy, active, and stress-free life. These symptoms have been isolated in our practice after working with many patients over decades. Repeatedly, we have proven Hiatal Hernia Syndrome to be the root cause of each and every one of them.

Yet, should you ask your primary care provider or gastroenterologist if your symptoms (such as heart palpitations, anxiety, shortness of breath, fatigue and more) are caused by your hiatal hernia, your doctor will assure you they are not.

Why don't they appreciate the connection between the long list of symptoms we have reviewed and Hiatal Hernia Syndrome? Your doctor simply has not been trained in Hiatal Hernia Syndrome.

The larger problem is covered in CHAPTER 1: INTRODUCTION TO ROOT CAUSE MEDICINE. In it we review the almost one-hundred-and-eighty-degree difference in diagnostic and treatment methodology between conventional medicine and root cause medicine.

Your hiatal hernia is most likely being diagnosed by a gastroenterologist. To think that a specialist trained only in digestive function would make the connection between your hiatal hernia and symptoms affecting your heart, lungs, and hormonal function – to name a few – is asking the gastroenterologist to think in a way he or she has not been trained.

Specialists are highly compartmentalized. If your journey with Hiatal Hernia Syndrome has already included a visit to the E.R. due to heart palpitations, shortness of breath or anxiety, you have likely been evaluated for a heart attack or any abnormality of your heart or lungs. And you have likely been "cleared" of any disease process.

Therefore, cardiologists and pulmonologists have already "excused you" as a patient. You do not have heart or lung disease, so they have said goodbye.

Now the gastroenterologist reviews the findings of the other specialists and all that he can offer is a medication for your reflux.

This scenario likely sounds familiar.

Let us not forget the potential presence of anxiety or panic attacks. Is any doctor going to appreciate the true root cause as Hiatal Hernia Syndrome? Not in the conventional medicine model. Instead, you will be ushered to a psychologist, psychiatrist, or perhaps even your PCP (primary care physician), who will suggest psychiatric medication for you, since they can find no other reason for your anxiety or panic attacks.

Why? They "know" there is no association between your anxiety and your acid reflux, therefore psychiatric medication is the only option, in their opinion. They are wrong in this assumption. Remember, their goal is to mask symptoms, not get to the root cause of them.

Most of my Hiatal Hernia Syndrome patients have had experiences similar to what we have just described. To call it "frustrating" is a gross understatement. It is positively maddening.

If you heard some of the stories from patients who have suffered for many years (sometimes more than ten) with this condition, your heart would go out to them. Some have lost the ability to lead a normal life. Some suffer so much anxiety they have had to go on disability, unable to make a living. The stories are very sad.

You may be such a sufferer. For all the time you have been suffering with no real help, We are sorry; we know how miserable it can be.

For myself and my team, the lack of proper and effective treatment you have been offered is inexcusable. It is what drives us to educate you and others about the true nature of this syndrome and your options for safe, non-drug-based and effective treatment.

We often wonder how long it will be before accurate awareness of this syndrome occurs. We do not hold out much hope unfortunately, because our conventional medicine model is completely symptom- and drug-based.

Hiatal Hernia Syndrome does not respond to drugs. That is not where the success in treatment lies, and it is for that reason we do not expect there to be any changes in what doctors will recommend when they diagnose a small or sliding hiatal hernia.

It is for this reason that the root cause approach provides the hopeful solution so lacking in the sea of misdiagnosis and ineffective treatment offered by conventional medicine. It is this lack of effective treatment that prompted the writing of this book.

It has been so disheartening to witness how hiatal hernia can completely derail the lives of those suffering. We have seen this firsthand: the mom who can no longer care for her children, the dad who has lost his job, the young person who no longer has any friends because no one understands why he feels the way he does.

Those who have been lucky enough to find out about our program have done well, but those people amount to a very small percentage of the overall sufferers; the true scale of the suffering and debilitation is vast.

We are hopeful this book will be shared, and it will provide hope and information to those who need it such that we can truly make inroads in widespread effective treatment.

CHAPTER 10

WHY IS HIATAL HERNIA SYNDROME UNDIAGNOSED OR MISDIAGNOSED?

There are really two problems that speak to why the syndrome is so frequently misdiagnosed or completely undiagnosed.

Difficulty in diagnosis

Unless the hiatal hernia is very pronounced, it evades the standard diagnostic procedures of either upper endoscopy, barium X-ray, or less commonly, esophageal manometry.

The upper endoscopy involves your doctor inserting a thin, flexible tube that is equipped with a camera (the endoscope) down your throat, to allow for the examination of your esophagus and stomach. From this test it will be determined if there is inflammation in either location.

It will typically rule out the presence of a bacterium called Helicobacter pylori (H. pylori), and if your stomach has risen above the level of the opening between it and your esophagus, a hiatal hernia will be diagnosed. You may also be told of the presence of ulcers, gastritis, polyps and more.

A barium X-ray is a special type of X-ray taken after you drink a liquid that coats the inside of your digestive tract. The coating will allow your doctor to visualize a silhouette of your esophagus, stomach, and upper small intestine.

Esophageal manometry is a test that utilizes high resolution to measure the function of the sphincter or valve between your esophagus and stomach. This valve, when functioning properly, prevents reflux or the backwards flow of stomach acid into your esophagus. This test is good at evaluating if your esophagus is able to move food properly into your stomach and if the valve is functioning correctly.

We have had many patients who have had more than one of the above diagnostic tests only to have one "show" a hiatal hernia while another one finds nothing. It can be confusing, especially when the end result is that your doctor can offer no assistance for your chronic symptoms.

A 2017 study from European Surgery gave some clarity as to why patients frequently report that one form of testing showed a hiatal hernia while another did not[6].

---

6   Eur Surg. 2017; 49(5): 210–217. Published online 2017 Sep 19. doi: 10.1007/s10353-017-0492-y *"Preoperative diagnosis of hiatal hernia: barium swallow X-ray, high-resolution manometry, or endoscopy?"* Michael Weitzendorfer, MD, et al.

Analyzing 112 patients, the researchers showed no correlation between the barium swallow X-ray and either an endoscope or esophageal manometry. There was, however, nice correlation between the endoscope and manometry.

When evaluating a correlation with GERD, or acid reflux, only the endoscopy showed a correlation with demonstrating the presence of hiatal hernia. Likely, this is why endoscopy is most often used when patients complain of GERD. No correlation could be found with barium swallow X-ray or esophageal manometry.

The researchers felt that esophageal manometry offered advantages over other testing methods with its ability to identify obstruction, motility problems and hiatal hernia itself.

We thought it was interesting that they discussed a lack of clarity as to which position was best for the test: supine (lying on your back) or standing. This particular team of researchers "split the difference" and used the supine position but combined it with a thirty-degree upper body elevation.

This elevation is similar to what you may have been advised to use at night to reduce reflux. Those who suffer often find some relief with elevating the head of their bed or sleeping on a wedge, although the latter is often disruptive to sleep for other reasons, mostly to do with comfort.

Gravity, of course, helps to hold things down. The researchers made mention that a sliding hiatal hernia's detection might be lessened by the positioning of the patient. It only makes sense, and it answers the question of why patients are frequently more uncomfortable at night: lying down reduces the ability of gravity to hold your stomach down.

The researchers did see a correlation between the size of the hiatal hernia as measured by esophageal manometry and the presence of GERD as a symptom. The larger the hiatal hernia, the more common the correlation with GERD.

The team concluded that the highest rate of detection of hiatal hernia (76.8%) was found from the barium swallow X-ray. But given their druthers, they preferred all three be performed for "the reliable exclusion of hiatal hernia prior to treatment."

Of course, the research environment is very different from the patient and doctor interaction, where the number of tests, their cost, and insurance coverage all need to be considered. Clearly, the performing of all three testing procedures is not something your insurance company would condone.

Further discussion of their conclusions validated the "considerable variation" in the detection of hiatal hernia. There was decent correlation between endoscopy and manometry. However, when evaluating integrity of the valve between your stomach and esophagus (gastroesophageal flap valve), again the endoscopy was best. There was no good correlation with esophageal manometry nor X-ray. The barium swallow X-ray did not show a correlation to the esophageal manometry in terms of hiatal hernia detection or identifying an abnormal esophageal valve.

Clearly, we have no "perfect test" for hiatal hernia detection. We are referring to overt hiatal hernia in this context, not the sliding nor subclinical type, which we will discuss below in the section TYPES OF HIATAL HERNIAS.

Conventional doctors are untrained in Hiatal Hernia Syndrome and all its associated symptoms

Doctors are not trained on the variety of symptoms associated with hiatal hernias. Traditional medicine has a narrow view of hiatal hernia:

- It is an overt displacement of your stomach above your diaphragm
- If it is very large, surgery is the treatment
- If it is not large, palliative treatment of symptoms, typically antacids, are prescribed.

That is it. Those three points encompass the complete evaluation of hiatal hernia.

It is hard to "blame" them for not understanding something they were never educated about.

Except... Why don't they pay attention to their patients? After all, we and our team were not trained on it either. But we do listen to our patients and we diagnose from a root cause viewpoint, and from this we began to notice a definite pattern in our patients.

How many patients would you need to see with acid reflux or GERD that ALSO complained of shortness of breath, heart palpitations, panic attacks, anxiety, constipation, burping, etc., etc., before you would begin to wonder what was going on?

How many patients would you need to meet who shared their story of panic attacks or anxiety that had never occurred before their digestive problems began?

How many patients would need to tell you they are not really the "anxious" or "depressed" type, yet their panic attack scared the heck out of them, and they have no idea why they are now chronically suffering?

We put it together. The pattern emerged for us, and the success of our treatment gave us all the validation we needed. Clearly the symptoms were related and thus was born "Hiatal Hernia Syndrome," a form of hiatal hernia that involved many other parts of the body to create a long list of symptoms that were quite debilitating.

Sadly, the conventional medicine approach to these patients should not be surprising. We refer you back to CHAPTER 1: INTRODUCTION TO ROOT CAUSE MEDICINE, in which we review the difference in how we think about the human body and its ability to heal itself, as opposed to the conventional medicine mindset that prefers to manage your symptoms with drugs.

Types of Hiatal Hernias

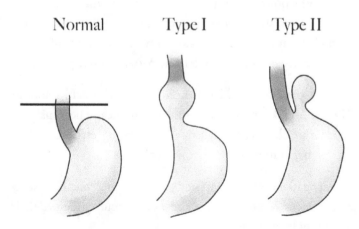

Normal   Type I   Type II

Any type of herniation of the stomach into the chest (meaning above your diaphragm) is a hiatal hernia. The herniation occurs through the hole or hiatus in the diaphragm through which the esophagus passes.

Your mouth is connected to your stomach via the tube called an esophagus. Your esophagus normally extends below the diaphragm about two to four centimeters. This means the sphincter separating your esophagus from your stomach is normally that distance below your diaphragm.

The diaphragm demarcates your chest from your abdomen. Your heart and lungs are in your chest, while your stomach, along with the rest of your digestive system and several other organs, all reside in your abdomen.

The take-away point is that your stomach is designed to be located beneath your diaphragm in your abdomen.

Type I

The most common is the sliding hiatal hernia, also known as type I. This type accounts for about ninety-five percent of all the hiatal hernias diagnosed and is the one most associated with the development of GERD.

In a sliding hiatal hernia, the lower part of your esophagus and stomach slide up into your chest through the diaphragm. (Such movement is normally prevented by the sphincter between your stomach and esophagus.) As a result of this hernia, it is very common for stomach acid to leak out into your esophagus, leading to the development of GERD.

Sliding hiatal hernias are typically designated as small, or mild, and are diagnosed during an endoscopy or X-ray. Despite identifying them, many doctors will not mention their presence to you, the patient. Why? They do not believe the condition causes any symptoms. Sadly, they are very much mistaken.

A sliding hiatal hernia is given its name because it can move up, inappropriately, above the diaphragm and back down below it. Due to this movement, your doctor may fail to "catch" it. This means you can have the problem of a sliding hiatal hernia that is completely missed during your X-ray or scope because at the time the test was performed, all appeared normal.

Some of the factors leading to a false negative are:

- The position you are in during the endoscopy. Most often the patient is in a partially seated position which allows gravity to "help" keep the stomach down.

- Tests are done with you fasting; an empty stomach is less likely to be elevated.

- Your level of constipation can affect the test. If you have recently "cleaned out" your colon, there is less intra-abdominal pressure and you are less likely to show elevation of the stomach.

Type II

The paraesophageal hiatal hernia, also known as type II, is considered to account for less than five percent of all hiatal hernias. A 2015 journal article from JAMA Surgery stated the incidence was up to ten percent as our population ages[7].

---

7   JAMA Network *"Long-term Quality of Life and Risk Factors for Recurrence After Laparoscopic Repair of Paraesophageal Hernia"* Anne O. Lidor, MD, MPH1;

Paraesophageal hernias are less common but yield the greatest number of complications. In this hernia the stomach herniates, or moves up, through the diaphragmatic esophageal hiatus up alongside the esophagus. It creates a dramatically enlarged opening and puts the stomach at increased risk due to strangulation or loss of blood flow to the stomach itself. If more than thirty percent of the stomach herniates into the chest it is called a giant paraesophageal hernia and surgery is required.

"Pure" type II hernias are rare.

Type III

This type of hiatal hernia is a combination of types I and II. Not only is the junction between the stomach and esophagus (gastroesophageal junction) herniated above the diaphragm, but the stomach is also herniated alongside the esophagus.

Most paraesophageal hernias are type III, though both type II and type III hernias are rare, together accounting for only five percent of all diagnosed hiatal hernias.

When both the stomach and esophagus are above the diaphragm, stomach acid entering the esophagus is not the problem, but hernia strangulation is. A strangulated hernia is one where the blood supply has been cut off to a particular tissue, typically the stomach in this case. As the tissue loses blood supply it releases toxins into your bloodstream which can lead to sepsis, a medical emergency that can be life-threatening. Fortunately, this is a very rare occurrence.

When surgery is required, the surgeon will pull the stomach down

Kimberley E. Steele, MD1; Miloslawa Stem, MS1; et al

below the diaphragm and sew up the enlarged opening. Unfortunately, the success rate of this surgery is quite poor. It makes sense that it would be, considering they are not addressing the underlying cause of the problem.

Per Anne O. Lidor MD, author of a published research article, "repair of paraesophageal hernias can be technically challenging". Due to this difficulty and the tendency for poor outcomes, surgery is typically reserved for those with life-threatening complications.

Dr. Lidor notes that while it is often cited that surgical repair can be safe, with minimal post-operative risk, "these reports are limited to short-term follow-up". There is little data regarding long-term function and quality of life. She further notes a disappointingly high recurrence rate of more than fifty percent following laparoscopic surgery[8].

Type IV

This type of hiatal hernia is quite rare. Personally, we have never seen one. In type IV, not just the stomach, but other abdominal organs such as the small intestine, spleen, and colon, have also herniated into the chest. The literature says this type can occur without symptoms, which we find hard to believe. But keep in mind they say that about all hiatal hernias. The flaw of such reasoning is what prompted the writing of this book.

---

8   JAMA Network "*Long-term Quality of Life and Risk Factors for Recurrence After Laparoscopic Repair of Paraesophageal Hernia*" Anne O. Lidor, MD, MPH1; Kimberley E. Steele, MD1; Miloslawa Stem, MS1; et al

"Subclinical hiatal hernia"

We would like to proffer an additional type of hiatal hernia: we call it type 0, or a subclinical hiatal hernia. It is defined as a condition whereby the stomach is spasmed, inappropriately pushing upward on your diaphragm, exerting stress on the esophageal sphincter.

This type can also involve an elevation of your diaphragm, similar to what I've just described with the spasmed stomach. It creates stress on the esophageal sphincter due to the inappropriate elevation of the stomach and/or diaphragm. It appears that just a slight amount of diaphragm displacement is all that is required to initiate the diaphragmatic spasm.

Type 0 is less severe than type I, but based on our clinical experience, no less symptomatic. Here at Root Cause Medical Clinic we have found it capable of creating some or all of the symptoms we've discussed. We see this type 0 often and, based on its ability to create a host of miserable symptoms, it deserves to be acknowledged as its own unique type of hiatal hernia in my opinion.

Type 0 is the most subtle of all the hiatal hernia types, but it has been validated that bigger does not mean worse.

You would assume that the larger the hiatal hernia, the worse the symptoms. This is not the case in our clinical experience. An older research paper from American Surgeon corroborates our findings.

Researcher C.J. Donald and team published a study evaluating eighty-three cases of hiatal hernia[9]; they noted that the size of the hernia is no indication of the severity of symptoms. In fact, some of the small hernias – barely recognizable on X-ray or endoscopy – can

---

9   Donald, C.J., et al., *"Diaphragmatic hernia: A report of eighty-three cases"*, American Surgeon, Vol 21 (1955)

cause the most severe symptoms. Meanwhile more "significant" hernias may be completely asymptomatic.

Dr. Donald and his team further noted that hernia can cause pressure on the heart, resulting in palpitations and tachycardia (rapid heartbeat). As we all know, heart disease is the number one killer of all Americans.

Due to the causal relationship of hiatal hernia affecting the heart, the report encouraged that in all hiatal hernia cases a differential diagnosis must be made to rule out any heart complications.

If you have visited an E.R. or Urgent Care in the past, you have likely experienced a thorough cardiac work-up, only to be told your heart is fine. What fails to occur is the ruling out of a hiatal hernia. You can have one condition without the other, or both at the same time. A proper diagnosis is critical.

Although a hiatal hernia can affect the heart – creating palpitations and rapid heart rate – EKGs are unaffected. Hence your "normal" heart work-up.

Hopefully, the data contained in this chapter explains why Hiatal Hernia Syndrome is so woefully misdiagnosed or undiagnosed, leading to avoidable suffering.

Next, we move on to Treatment.

CHAPTER 11

TREATMENT OF HIATAL HERNIA SYNDROME, CONVENTIONAL VS. ROOT CAUSE MEDICINE

Regarding treatment, we would like to begin with the conventional medicine approach to the treatment of hiatal hernia.

Conventional medicine approach

If you look online, the Mayo Clinic says: "Most people with a hiatal hernia don't experience any signs or symptoms and won't need treatment. If you experience signs and symptoms, such as recurrent heartburn and acid reflux, you may need medication or surgery."

Stanford Health Care offers three options for care:

1. Diet and lifestyle change. Specifically, they mention that losing weight and reducing alcohol consumption may help "manage acid reflux symptoms". They are not wrong, but it is certainly providing no specifics for the individual suffering.

2. Medications. It is stated that if diet and lifestyle changes are not effective, then medications to treat GERD should be considered.

3. Surgery. If none of the above work, surgery is recommended.

You can look in vain for any information from the conventional medicine arena that suggests a symptomatic profile of anything other than GERD.

They do acknowledge some symptoms secondary to GERD, such as chest discomfort produced by the acid reflux, pressure of the stomach on the diaphragm, and difficulty swallowing, but again it is all acid reflux related.

A recent study epitomizes the "blinders" to anything but acid reflux as relates to hiatal hernia. In the 2019 study published in *Medicine Pharmacy Reports* titled "*The management of hiatal hernia: an update on diagnosis and treatment10*" led by researcher Alice Sfara, she notes that it is a common condition in the general population, frequently caused by increased intra-abdominal pressure.

The risk factors are noted as: being overweight or elderly, history of multiple pregnancies, esophageal surgery, or any structural abnormalities.

---

10 Reference: MPR Medicine Pharmacy Reports "*The management of hiatal hernia: an update on diagnosis and treatment*" Alice Sfara and Dan L. Dumitrascu

Dr. Sfara relates the symptoms as due to acid reflux. She states classic symptoms include regurgitation and heartburn, with less common symptoms including dysphagia (trouble swallowing), epigastric pain (above the stomach), chest pain, and even chronic iron deficiency anemia.

The goal, she states, is to reduce the symptoms of gastroesophageal reflux disease (GERD) by addressing gastric acid secretion.

Everything is focused on acid reflux and how to "handle" it; there is no mention of any "reason or cause" of the acid reflux, and how to address it.

Lifestyle modifications are the first line of defense, including such measures as:

- Weight loss
- Elevating the head of the bed
- Avoidance of meals two to three hours before bedtime
- Elimination of "trigger" foods such as chocolate, alcohol, caffeine, spicy foods, citrus, carbonated drinks.

We would like to differentiate between trigger foods and causative foods. Trigger foods will aggravate or exacerbate the already inflamed esophagus or stomach.

Causative foods are at the root of why it all began.

Reducing trigger foods is helpful in reducing symptoms, but they are not the root cause of the problem.

We want to heal the problem, not just reduce the aggravation of it. More on that later in this chapter.

Continuing with the results of this study: if the lifestyle changes are insufficient, the next step is the administration of drugs. The author quotes what the American College of Gastroenterology recommends, which is an eight-week course of PPIs as the therapy of choice for GERD symptom relief.

Dr. Sfara states "the current recommendation is to use the minimal dose of PPI that is sufficient to control symptoms."

That sounds good: a two-month course might not create too much damage. But if you are a patient who has been through this type of regimen then you know that it very rarely stops after eight weeks unless you yourself demand it. Often, patients who experience no relief, or who experience side effects they find miserable, will discontinue the medications. Other times their doctor will offer a different type of antacid or proton pump inhibitor, all designed to lessen acid production.

However, even when they do provide relief, we frequently meet patients who have maintained their dose over the course of years, not weeks. This is dangerous and they are not told of the side effects that can create long-term ill health, such as bone weakening and an unhealthy digestive tract.

It is ironic that the drug is prescribed to "help" a digestive malfunction, yet its long-term use only worsens digestive health. That is a fact most patients are not made aware of by their doctor.

Again, surgical intervention was recommended in this study if the above measures are unsuccessful.

There you have it. The results and recommendations of this study, along with those of Mayo Clinic and Stanford Health Center, pretty well sum up the conventional medicine viewpoint and treatment recommendations.

What are the commonly recommended medications?

Common medications for either heartburn or reflux include the following.

Antacids that neutralize stomach acid

Common over-the-counter options are Mylanta, Rolaids, and Tums, which may provide quick (though temporary) relief.

Overuse of some antacids can cause side effects such as diarrhea, constipation, and stomach cramps. These products all contain calcium, potentially putting you at risk of kidney stones and constipation.

Medications to reduce acid production

Known as H2 receptor blockers, common names include cimetidine (Tagamet), famotidine (Pepcid), and ranitidine (Zantac*). These are available over the counter plus stronger versions are available by prescription from your doctor.

> *Note: As of this writing, Zantac was recently removed from the market due to the presence of the contaminant NDMA (N-Nitrosodimethylamine), a probable human carcinogen. What is most concerning – over and above the fact that it has been investigated for at least two years, beginning in 2018, and only just was banned – is that the drug has been in production for thirty-nine years. It was first launched in 1981 and became the world's best-selling drug by 1987. All drugs have side effects, and you should be very wary of taking any, but we have always been particularly concerned with "new" drugs whose true side effects remain unknown for several years. Zantac was far

from being a new drug, yet it has now been banned due to a cancer-causing contaminant.

What types of cancers is NDMA linked to? Sadly, the list is ridiculously long, encompassing almost every major organ you possess. Ironically, it includes both esophageal and stomach cancers, the very organs one is supposedly trying to protect with the use of antacids.

List of cancers associated with NDMA:

- Stomach
- Esophagus
- Small intestine
- Large intestine
- Kidney
- Bladder
- Liver (even small amounts of NDMA have been linked to liver toxicity)
- Pancreas
- Prostate
- Leukemia
- Non-Hodgkin's lymphoma
- Multiple myeloma

The contaminant or impurity increases in potency over time, and when stored at higher than normal room temperatures. The FDA tested many, many samples before they made the connection. However, they found that tablets of Zantac that were neither "old" nor stored at temperatures higher than "room temperature" still contained the contaminant.

Zantac's pedigree was impressive: it became the world's best-selling drug and one of the first to ever top one billion dollars in annual sales. (Underscore "annual" sales of a billion dollars.)

As a final word on NDMA, you should know that the contaminant has also been detected in several blood pressure medications, including valsartan, losartan, and irbesartan. These drugs, known as "-sartan" drugs, are amongst a class of medicines called angiotensin II receptor blocker (ARBs). They are used to treat high blood pressure and heart failure. If you're taking them or know anyone who is, please consult your doctor to speak about alternatives, or better yet consult a functional medicine doctor to see what can be done about getting to the root cause of your high blood pressure. Here at Root Cause Medical Clinics we have excellent success getting our patients off their blood pressure medication once the root cause has been treated.

Returning to the group of medications of which Zantac is a part (H2 blockers), the known side effects include:

- Constipation
- Diarrhea
- Nausea
- Vomiting
- Headache
- Difficulty sleeping
- Dry mouth
- Dry skin
- Ringing in the ears
- A runny nose

Medications that block acid production (also designed to heal the esophagus)

These are known as proton pump inhibitors. They are stronger acid blockers than the H2 receptor blockers we just discussed. Their strong effects are aimed at giving your damaged esophageal lining time to heal.

Over-the-counter proton pump inhibitors include lansoprazole (Prevacid 24HR) and omeprazole (Prilosec, Losec, Zegerid). Even stronger versions are available with a prescription from your doctor.

The most common side effects of proton pump inhibitors are:

- Headache
- Diarrhea
- Constipation
- Abdominal pain
- Flatulence
- Fever
- Vomiting
- Nausea
- Rash

If you have been on a PPI for a while, you were likely told by your doctor that the drug is very well tolerated, and side effects are rare.

Also, providing the overt side effects have not been too bothersome, you've likely been on the drug for more than a year. We frequently meet patients who have been taking a PPI for several years, sometimes longer than a decade.

If you are in this category, you will likely find this next section concerning. Even if you have just started taking the medication, please heed the following data.

The "safety profile" for PPIs has not held up to recent scrutiny. More serious side effects include:

- Chronic kidney disease
- Fracture, increased risk of bone fractures
- Infections
- Clostridium difficile diarrhea – a potentially life-threatening condition
- Pneumonia
- Dementia
- Vitamin and mineral deficiencies – including B12 and magnesium

It is stated that these side effects are "rare" and generally **associated with long-term use**.

Please note the drug manufacturer's definition of "long-term use": **Using the products for more than a year!**

As we mentioned, we regularly meet patients who have been taking their PPI for several years who have not been counseled on the dangers of having done so.

There is a rebound phenomenon that you should be aware of if you have been taking a PPI for a while. The "rebound" involves an increase of stomach acid production above the level present before taking the drug. It is believed to be a mechanism whereby the long-term suppression of acid production from the medication results in a rebound increase above normal levels after discontinuing the drug.

Of course, this results in even worse heartburn or acid reflux, causing you to seek out your doctor once again for assistance. This "reinforcing loop" (as the authors of this study from 2019[11] refer to it), creates such a dependency that successful weaning from antacids can prove to be near impossible.

Anxiety and Depression Medications

As we have discussed, the long list of symptoms associated with Hiatal Hernia Syndrome include many that are emotionally based. Anxiety and depression are common. Unfortunately, conventional medicine does not seek out their root cause, but rather masks them with dangerous psychotropic drugs after giving you a diagnosis of panic attacks, anxiety, or depression.

Based on thousands of cases we have evaluated, it is rare that an individual suffering from Hiatal Hernia Syndrome has not been prescribed a psychotropic drug. These drugs are ineffective, have life-threatening side effects and only serve to complicate the problem with new drug-induced symptoms.

Root Cause Treatment of Hiatal Hernia Syndrome

In this section we will share with you how we treat Hiatal Hernia Syndrome here at Root Cause Medical Clinic. Keep in mind: there are close to twenty different symptoms that individuals with this problem can experience. Some are "classic" like heartburn, others are less common.

---

11   Reference: MedSafe publication "*Proton pump inhibitors and rebound acid hypersecretion – A recurring issue*"

The basics are these:

1. Hiatal Hernia Syndrome is very common.

2. Hiatal Hernia Syndrome has the potential to cause a vast array of symptoms, most of which your medical professional will assure you have nothing to do with the problem.

3. Too often patients are told their legitimate Hiatal Hernia Syndrome symptoms are "all in their head" or that "they are symptoms that cannot be treated and simply need to be put up with."

Our clinical experience with the above put us on the path of becoming experts in this area.

The Root Cause Medicine approach stems from some basic principles:

- The body is designed to function optimally.
- The body has an underlying reason for all the symptoms it creates.
- If we can unburden the body sufficiently, it will heal.

It is the above knowledge that gives us our tenacity to carry on.

It is that knowledge that leads to our success.

You have read some of the success stories included in this book. For every one of those, how many tens or hundreds of thousands of men and women are suffering needlessly, having their lives ruined by this condition?

How many are being "treated" with dangerous psychiatric drugs, putting them at risk of life-threatening side effects?

It was out of the concern of so much needless suffering that we wrote this book. We had to share the knowledge that we, as a team, have amassed while treating hundreds of patients over decades.

Treatment of Hiatal Hernia Syndrome is a very personal and individualized journey.

The question we need to answer for you is: how did you get here and how can we reverse it?

It is also important to appreciate that for each patient, more than one cause can be present.

The major root cause of Hiatal Hernia Syndrome is an elevated stomach and/or diaphragm, potentially in spasm. They have become pushed upward, often compromising the ability of the valve between your stomach and esophagus to function correctly.

The above is often the "start" of obvious symptoms, but in order to truly correct it we need to understand why it occurred, and that underlying problem may have been present for years.

Successful treatment for Hiatal Hernia Syndrome involves treating the root cause of why the diaphragm cannot maintain its normal strength and tone. We also need to discover what created sufficient pressure on the stomach and within your abdomen to push the stomach up – and sometimes through – the diaphragm.

Treatment involves both internal, nutritional and structural care. Typically, each type of care is part of a hiatal hernia program. Occasionally, it is just one or the other, but we are going to review all the possible care options below.

Internal Medicine Treatment

We approach the problem by evaluating and treating the cause of increased pressure in the abdomen. The pressure can be caused by:

- Poor diet
- Food sensitivities
- Bacterial or parasitic infection
- Yeast overgrowth
- Virus overload
- Toxins
- Excessive gas and bloating
- Constipation
- Incomplete digestion of foods
- Malabsorption
- Nutrient deficiencies
- Imbalanced microbiome or dysbiosis
- Weakened abdominal muscles, including those muscles around the diaphragm
- Nerve irritation

The last two areas are evaluated by our Physical Medicine Department, consisting of our Doctor of Physical Therapy and Doctor of Chiropractic.

There can be an inter-relationship between these, as you will see during the discussion of each below.

We utilize many tools, as needed, for our individualized programs.

We want to review – in order of commonality – the treatments we use to successfully address Hiatal Hernia Syndrome.

Diet Change

Since it most often begins within the digestive tract, it should not surprise you to learn that we frequently find a dietary component associated with hiatal hernias. After all, what goes into the stomach? Food!

As mentioned earlier, a person who is eating a poor diet – or eating something they are reacting to – can suffer a hiatal hernia. Realize the individual may not even have indigestion, but what they are eating is still the cause of the stomach and/or diaphragm spasm.

If you consume a food (or drink) you are sensitive to, your stomach can react by going into spasm or moving upward. Food sensitivities (not allergies, which are different) are a very common cause of hiatal hernia.

Food sensitivities can be tricky to identify. Certainly, if every time you drank milk you got acid reflux, you would have figured out the association. But food sensitivities are unlike allergies, which do tend to have a fast response. Food sensitivities can have a delayed reaction time, making them elusive to an obvious diagnosis for the patient.

What is different about our treatment is that it is the personalized approach. It is all very well and good to tell someone not to eat spicy foods, citrus, caffeine, or chocolate – known irritants to an already inflamed stomach. It is something else to determine exactly WHY the problem developed in the first place.

This is where the detection of food sensitivities comes in. We find it interesting to note that the true root cause of stomach inflammation and resultant acid reflux, food-wise, is very different from the exacerbators of symptoms. What we mean is that common food sensitivities are gluten and dairy, while common exacerbators are the above-mentioned spicy foods, citrus, etc. Gluten and dairy are the two most common food sensitivities, yet they are "bland" foods, certainly not spicy, and ironically, they are often recommended "to settle" an upset stomach.

Gluten can also cause swelling of the small intestine, exacerbating your symptoms of Hiatal Hernia Syndrome.

A big "miss" by conventional medicine is their focus on managing symptoms vs. isolating and identifying root causes.

Food sensitivities are a key example of this. Accurate identification of a food sensitivity often puts an end to acid reflux. This is a common result for our patients here at Root Cause Medical Clinic.

We use a Root Cause modified elimination diet to help us identify food sensitivities. Elimination diets remain the gold standard for identifying any food sensitivities you may suffer from.

You may be thinking: "Isn't there a blood test I can do?" There are delayed sensitivity IgG blood tests designed to identify food sensitivities. They sound so great: give a little blood and get analyzed for two hundred different foods.

We believe one day these tests will be accurate, and that will be a happy day; it will make life much easier. But as of right now these tests are riddled with false positives, and it is for that reason we use them very infrequently.

We have tried many, but we keep coming back to the gold standard of the elimination diet, which is tried and true. There is a great blood test for gluten, but other than that test, the rest of the food sensitivities are best identified through the elimination diet, which, after the elimination process, follows up with provocation of foods in a systematic fashion.

Once food sensitivities are successfully identified and removed from your diet, your stomach's irritation is reduced considerably. It therefore stops spasming and relaxes to such a degree that it stops "squirting" acid up into your esophagus. Your esophagus heals and you are back to enjoying citrus and spicy foods, provided you enjoyed them before. You must continue to avoid the food you are sensitive to, however – sometimes permanently.

Infections

Infections are a common culprit of Hiatal Hernia Syndrome. They can cause bloating, swelling and irritation of the lining of the intestine, not to mention weakening your immune system. Therefore, treatment includes evaluating your body for bacteria, parasites, yeast, fungi, and viruses. A medical endoscopy typically assesses only for the H. pylori bacterial infection of the stomach; other infections are missed because they are not even considered.

Even H. pylori, once identified, is not followed up well once it is identified.

Treatment for H. pylori is a "brutal" trio of antibiotics plus ant-acids. Some patients do not even complete treatment because it is too miserable. (From Dr. Vikki: I personally went through it many years ago. I was healthy and it was found incidentally, yet I struggled with how much upset it caused in my digestive tract.)

We have since created a protocol that is still efficacious, but much less harsh than the standard medical protocol.

What some patients do not realize is the importance of completing the treatment, along with the necessity of retesting to ensure the bacteria is eradicated.

It is also unappreciated that you can contract the infection again. One treatment does not confer lifetime immunity.

H. pylori is a bacterium that can destroy the acid-producing cells in your stomach, while at the same time giving you symptoms of excess acid. It is a classic example of why managing symptoms alone is a dangerous proposition.

Missing the presence of H. pylori can potentially cause permanent damage to your stomach.

There are other infectious agents including bacteria, fungi, parasites, and yeast that can all cause inflammation within your digestive tract. Identifying their presence and taking the correct steps to eliminate them is crucial.

SIBO (small intestinal bacterial overgrowth) is not an infection, but we include it in this section because it involves the presence of bacteria that are normal to your gut, but are residing in the wrong area i.e. your small intestine. So, while SIBO is not something you "catch," like H. pylori, it does involve the inappropriate growth of bacteria that should only be present lower in your intestine. It can cause digestive pain, diarrhea, bloating and lead to the increased intra-abdominal pressure we know to be a root cause of Hiatal Hernia Syndrome.

The conventional medical treatment for SIBO involves treating the overgrowth with an expensive medication, rifaximin. Expense aside, the overgrowth tends to recur, and patients are prescribed the drug again.

If you tease it apart from a root cause lens, you will learn that bacteria entering your small intestine should be eliminated with proper acid production in your stomach, proper enzyme production by your pancreas, and proper bile production by your liver. If these three areas of your intestinal tract were doing their jobs, you would not suffer from any bacterial overgrowth.

Does it make sense then that the proper way to address the problem is at the root of it, rather than "managing symptoms" with drugs? We think so too.

It can be complex; we are not going to sugar-coat it. It is easy to say, "You have SIBO, so take rifaximin." But that does not address the cause and it does not leave you with a healthy intestine.

It takes a bit more work to diagnose which organ is working correctly, which one is not and what to do to restore normal function.

It is here that we shine, having functional medicine testing to hand that provides us the correct tools. There are several tests we utilize; a comprehensive stool analysis is chief amongst them. Please do not confuse the stool testing offered by conventional medicine with a comprehensive stool analysis. They are very different. Conventional medicine typically looks for two to three parasites only. The comprehensive stool analysis evaluates for parasites, bacteria, amoeba, fungi, good and bad bacteria of the microbiome and more.

Perhaps you need to take hydrochloric acid. Maybe it is pancreatic enzymes you need. Perhaps your liver is burdened with too many toxins and it needs to be unburdened.

Toxins is our next section.

The goal is to sufficiently unburden whatever area(s) we find, such that your body begins to function optimally again.

We rarely need to use drugs to handle infections, although occasionally an antibiotic might be required for something that is not successfully addressed with more natural measures.

Do you have a genetic "flaw" such that you will need to support a certain part of your body with a supplement? This is the field of nutritional genomics and it is a very exciting one. Mom and dad gave you your genes; perhaps what you inherited predisposes you to a weakness in a certain area. That is okay. Once the weak gene is identified, often all that is required is a little extra support from a natural nutrient for it function correctly.

What this means is that if your family is predisposed to a certain disease (one that is found heavily in your family tree), nutritional genomics opens the door to potentially preventing you from developing that disease.

Toxins

Toxins abound in our environment. The good news is that your body is designed to rid itself of toxins. The design is there, but that does not mean you are performing the activity successfully.

We have found that liver function, bile production and overall gut health will all be compromised if the toxic burden is overwhelming. Not to mention your immune system.

It is for this reason we test for a variety of toxins, based on your symptoms and health history. Some common ones are mold and heavy metals.

We have a treatment protocol that safely removes toxins without chelation (a chemical process in which a synthetic solution is injected into the bloodstream to remove heavy metals and/or minerals from the body). Chelation can take years and often creates a lot of negative symptoms.

The key to detoxification is that it will not occur correctly if the body is inflamed. Therefore, both must be evaluated and treated to ensure detoxification is successful.

Excessive gas and bloating

It is very difficult to describe how miserable bloating and gas is to someone who has never experienced it. Gas and bloating are responsible for the increased intra-abdominal pressure that pushes the stomach and diaphragm upwards.

We know it is a problem. The key is treating the root cause of it.

Increased gas and resulting bloating can arise from everything we have discussed so far, plus many of the items we have left to discuss. In other words, there is no single "gas-X" that handles this problem for everyone.

That does not mean it is difficult to address – quite the contrary. There just is not a single cause.

What can it be?

Some of the most common reasons are lack of proper digestive "juices". If your gas or bloat happens quickly after eating, low stomach acid or SIBO can be a cause.

Let us discuss low stomach acid in more detail. A symptom of low stomach acid is heartburn. This sounds counter-intuitive to be sure, but it has been well documented.

Hydrochloric acid (HCl) is an important gastric secretion that enables the body to break down proteins, activate important enzymes and hormones, and protect against bacterial overgrowth in the gut.

The reason for the association is as follows: low stomach acid results in decreased digestion because the hydrochloric acid secreted by your stomach enables you to break down proteins, along with activating enzymes and hormones. The presence of the acid also protects you against bacterial overgrowth in your gut from orally ingested pathogens.

When insufficient stomach acid exists, your food is not being properly broken down. It begins to ferment, resulting in bloating and gas production. This state causes pressure on the sphincter between your stomach and esophagus (the lower esophageal sphincter or LES). When it cannot close normally, acid reflux occurs.

Increasing your stomach acid production to a normal level improves digestion and removes the pressure on the sphincter, effectively handling your acid reflux. This is not "opinion." It is basic anatomy and physiology.

A paper in *Nutrition Review* in 2018[12] confirmed this fact. The authors noted that our ability to properly digest and absorb our nutrients declines with age and that decreased stomach acid is one of the most common age-related causes of faulty digestion.

One study[13] found thirty percent of adults over the age of sixty

---

12   Nutrition Review article *"Gastric Balance: Heartburn Not Always Caused by Excess Acid"*

13   Krasinski SD, Russell RM, Samloff IM, Jacob RA, Dallal GE, McGandy RB, Hartz SC. *"Fundic atrophic gastritis in an elderly population. Effect on*

suffering from little to no acid production while a second study[14] found up to forty percent of postmenopausal women to have no stomach acid secretions.

The article listed the following symptoms to be associated with low stomach acid:

- Heartburn
- Indigestion
- Bloating
- Burning
- Diarrhea
- Acne, as an adult
- Nutrient deficiencies – particularly B vitamins and minerals
- Chronic intestinal infections
- Undigested food in stool

Is this a factor in why increasing age is directly associated with increased Hiatal Hernia Syndrome? It makes sense.

There are other (non-digestive) conditions associated with low stomach acid, including allergies, asthma, and gallstones.

Note: Age is a factor, but it is not the only one. We see many young patients in their twenties suffering from

---

hemoglobin and several serum nutritional indicators" J Am Geriatr Soc. 1986 Nov;34(11):800-6

14   Grossman MI, Kirsner JB, Gillespie IE. *"Basal and histalog-stimulated gastric secretion in control subjects and in patients with peptic ulcer or gastric cancer"* Gastroenterology 1963;45:15-26.

Hiatal Hernia Syndrome with concurrent poor stomach acid production.

Natural remedies to increase stomach acid production

Betaine hydrochloride (HCl) is a readily available supplement that has a long history of safety. You should consult your clinician (preferably a Functional Medicine doctor who has experience) on how best to begin a protocol.

Pepsin is also considered a safe supplement and has been used with a good safety record, often in conjunction with betaine hydrochloride. Again, it is best to consult your clinician to decide if it makes sense (based on your symptoms) to include pepsin.

Gentian, from the root Gentiana lutea, has been used as a digestive aid for centuries. It contains two of the most bitter substances known, which act to stimulate saliva secretion and stomach acid production.

Gentian is one of the major active ingredients of Swedish bitters, an herbal tonic dating back to the 15th century. For those of you who enjoy a little history: the doctor who created the tonic (Dr. Clause Samst) was Swedish, although he created the bitters tonic from his position of Surgeon General for Simon Bolivar's army in Venezuela. The tonic, named Swedish bitters, helped the soldiers with a variety of tropical stomach ailments.

Bitters are made from a range of aromatic herbs, roots, bark, and fruit. The health benefits of bitters have been well documented to not only increase digestive secretions, such as stomach acid, but to improve the absorption of nutrients, increase bile secretion by the liver, and boost peristalsis, a pattern of muscle contractions in the intestines that propels your food from your esophagus down through your intestines, ensuring normal absorption.

There is a family of alcoholic beverages called digestifs which simply take the botanicals and infuse them into flavorless alcohol. As their name suggests, digestifs were designed to be imbibed before a meal to enhance digestion. There were a variety of brands in wide use prior to Prohibition, which banned the use of any alcohol. Most brands disappeared at that time.

Some common alcoholic drinks containing bitters include the classic Old Fashioned and Manhattan. We are not proponents of drinking hard alcohol, but as a historical note we find it fascinating that the use of bitters has a long history.

You can enjoy all the benefits of bitters without any alcohol; we have seen excellent success in the use of bitters with our patients. The blend of botanicals makes them very palatable.

Peppermint is an herb that aids digestion through promoting the production of stomach acid. It also has antibacterial properties. It aids digestion by combating gas production, increases the flow of bile from your liver and has healing properties.

Peppermint is also an antispasmodic, found to decrease the tone of the esophagus sphincter, thus allowing the easier escape of air. This can relieve discomfort formed by spasms of the upper digestive tract.

Bloating that happens an hour or more after eating is more often linked to low pancreatic enzymes. When we address the normalization of your digestive function, the gas and bloat go away. It feels great!

Constipation

Getting to the root of constipation is, fortunately, something we find very easy. If you have suffered for years, do not worry: we have a high success rate.

Yes, it is multi-factorial. Is it food related? Often, yes. Is it from low fiber? It can be, and that is a common deficiency in the U.S., but we have certainly met our share of patients who were eating great quantities of fiber yet still suffered.

Is it dehydration? Again, this is a common deficiency amongst Americans, but it is not always the case.

What is the most common cause? What we see is food sensitivities, infections and toxins, plus the imbalance of the good bacteria of your gut, along with compromised functioning of your liver.

So again, it is a combination of factors.

Incomplete digestion of foods

Your digestive tract is beautifully designed. Digestion begins in your mouth with chewing. Your chewed food slides down your esophagus into a very acidic stomach that churns your food around and breaks it down into small particles. Your food then leaves your stomach, traveling into your small intestine where both bile and pancreatic enzymes get to work on continuing the digestive process.

The goal of digestion is to break food down into its component parts of carbohydrates, protein and fat, and have those elements cross out of your intestine into your bloodstream. Your blood then delivers the nutrients to your cells, where they eat.

The simplicity is that your body's organs and cells must be fed in order to perform their jobs correctly. If you cannot break down your food properly, it will not effectively feed your cells and organs.

When you suffer symptoms such as bloating, gas, constipation, acid reflux, GERD, diarrhea, etc., it is an indication of incomplete digestion of your food.

When you suffer from GERD, the barely digested food comes back up into your mouth. When you suffer from diarrhea, you may see incompletely digested food in your stool.

A body that is not breaking its food down correctly cannot function optimally.

Malabsorption

What we just discussed (incomplete digestion), holds true for malabsorption. They are very similar. Once food is broken down fully it needs to be absorbed into the bloodstream. Those who suffer with Hiatal Hernia Syndrome have an imbalance of their digestive tract that prevents optimal absorption.

It sounds counter-intuitive but when you suffer malabsorption, you will often tend to gain weight and have a big belly. You can be underweight too, but overweight is more common.

Nutrient deficiencies

As we have discussed, acid reflux and GERD are the most common symptoms associated with Hiatal Hernia Syndrome. We have also reviewed that antacids are the most common "treatment" prescribed.

While antacid medication can certainly make the symptoms of heartburn or GERD more comfortable, your stomach is designed to be a bag of acid for a reason. The acidic pH is what allows you to begin good digestion of food, plus it keeps bacteria and bad organisms from reproducing.

It becomes quite a vicious circle. Some patients have been on antacids for years, and it has set them up for malabsorption, maldigestion, infections and, as a result, worsening Hiatal Hernia Syndrome.

Certain nutrients are required to keep your GI tract healthy. The chronic use of antacids or other medications often deplete your body of the ability to absorb key nutrients.

We test for all the major nutrients and replace them, temporarily, while addressing the reason for the malabsorption. Once the root cause has been addressed, you typically will not need to continue supplementing.

Do note that a healthy, balanced diet comes into play here as well. If you are deficient because you rarely eat healthy fruits or vegetables and your diet lacks fiber, we will address that as well.

Imbalanced microbiome, or dysbiosis

Your microbiome is made up of a community of trillions of bacteria, viruses, and fungi. It is estimated you have about four times the number of organisms in your gut as you have cells in your body.

Dysbiosis refers to an imbalance of this community of organisms such that its healthy balance is no longer intact. Such an imbalance can be a cause of Hiatal Hernia Syndrome.

Causes of such imbalance are many. It can be due to a food

sensitivity, a poor diet, insufficient stomach acid, pancreatic enzymes, or improper bile flow. It can also be the result of taking certain medications.

Physical medicine treatments

The following series of treatments involves your physical body.

What we have reviewed so far has focused on restoring the function and balance of your digestive tract and other contributing internal organs and systems. This section focuses on the structural and neurological factors that also must be addressed, in most cases, to achieve a completely successful outcome.

Weakened muscles, including abdomen and those which affect the diaphragm

From a structural standpoint, weak abdominal muscles and a weakened core can put stress on the diaphragm, allowing it to ride upwards and flatten.

When functioning normally, the diaphragm muscles have a dome-like shape i.e. not flat. It is the flattening of the diaphragm that leads to the issues of malfunction that are so often seen in Hiatal Hernia Syndrome.

We utilize a comprehensive physical therapy assessment to determine if the diaphragm is functioning properly. If the diaphragm is spasmed it will be flattened, and the result is loss of the normal dome shape. The cascade of effects this causes is rather lengthy, as described below.

When you inhale, the diaphragm muscles bow downward, creating a vacuum effect that fills your large lungs with air. When you exhale, the reverse occurs: air is pushed upwards, creating a vacuum effect within the abdomen.

Diaphragmatic motion, therefore, goes beyond simple air flow. The normal functioning of the diaphragm affects circulation, your heart and digestive function. It is a lack of knowledge or appreciation of this interplay which, we believe, causes doctors to negate so many of the symptoms associated with this syndrome.

And remember, while you are alive your diaphragm never stops moving. When its motion is compromised to any degree, it starts to make sense that a myriad of problems can develop.

The loss of the dome shape inhibits the vacuum effect within the abdominal cavity, causing disturbances in how your food moves through your intestine and the efficiency of your digestion. Above the diaphragm, flattening affects the lungs. They are unable to expand fully, so air does not fully permeate the lower, deeper lobes of the lungs, creating hemodynamic problems (the dynamics of blood flow and circulation).

That is not all: flattening of the diaphragm also causes nerve problems. The vagus nerve and sympathetic nervous system are affected, causing the stress and panic attacks experienced by so many sufferers of the syndrome.

Lastly, flattening of the diaphragm causes the stomach to push up against it, leading to the classic herniation through the esophagus and the acid reflux or GERD.

Cause and effect go both ways. Not only does the flattening of the diaphragm affect the lungs, digestive and nervous system, but the reverse is true as well. Diaphragm flattening can be caused by lung malfunction, respiratory ailments, abdominal and digestive malfunction. All can lead to diaphragm flattening. Vagus nerve or sympathetic nervous system dysfunction can also lead to diaphragm flattening, as can poor core strength, diastasis recti (discussed earlier), and lastly, chronic low back and thoracic (middle back) pain.

It does not really matter which came first; the goal is to remedy the problem and try to ensure it does not recur.

Proper strength and balance of these muscles must be restored. This requires physical therapy treatment. It is called hands-on manual therapy, but not all physical therapists are adept at the treatment.

A proper physical therapy evaluation includes the following:

- Measuring the flexibility of your entire spine. Tightness, pain, and stiffness in the neck, middle back or lower back can indicate potential problems with rib cage function and muscle strength and can affect posture.

- Assessing the integrity and strength of all the muscles affecting your spine and diaphragm. There are many such muscles, including your upper traps, scapular muscles (those of the shoulder blade), psoas muscle (described in detail below), quadratus lumborum muscle, plus your abdominal or core muscles.

- Measuring muscle tone. Muscles can be overactive or underactive. Muscle spasms (an overactive state) are evaluated for along the lower rib cage and in your abdomen. With spasming can come a guarding reaction of the abdomen, neck or lower back, bloating, or a "rumbling" with palpation of the abdomen. Muscles cannot function properly if the nerve connecting to them is malfunctioning, therefore nerve evaluation is also part of a comprehensive evaluation, as you will see next.

- Nerve imbalance diagnosis, including the nerves in the neck, middle back, and lower back. The vagus nerve (a very important cranial nerve involved in Hiatal Hernia Syndrome) is also evaluated here. (We go into greater explanation of the vagus nerve in the next section.) Lastly, both balance and coordination are also part of this section.

- A measure of breathing circumference i.e. how much your chest expands when you take a deep breath. The physical therapist will utilize a tape measure to differentiate the circumference of your chest when you have exhaled and compare it to the measurement when you've fully inhaled. It is one of the metrics we use to assess your progress as you move through the program. We also assess your breathing rate (how often you normally take a breath).

- Posture assessment, with emphasis on your rib cage, the position of the pelvis (certain muscular imbalances will pull the pelvis out of its normal position), rounding of the middle back (kyphosis), curvature of the spine (scoliosis), forward position of the neck ("text neck").

- Palpation of the rib cage, diaphragm, middle back, and abdomen, looking for any discomfort, is another part of the comprehensive evaluation.

Once the evaluation is complete, treatment begins to address any abnormalities discovered.

Physical medicine treatments employ different modalities.

- Manual therapy is an important tool. There are many manual therapy techniques; they are performed by physical therapists to treat a variety of musculoskeletal pains or malfunctions.

Manual therapy involves manipulation of muscles and joints in very specific ways. To the untrained eye it could look like massage, however, if you are on the receiving end of treatment you are clear on the therapeutic difference. Hiatal Hernia Syndrome can require manual therapy of the diaphragm, rib cage, abdominal muscles, spine, and abdomen in the location of specific organs.

- Therapeutic exercises are also employed, including breathing techniques, posture correction, strengthening and stabilization of core and scapular muscles, plus pelvic floor training.

- Certain cases require a specialized treatment called vagus nerve balancing or vagus nerve reset. Some Doctors of Physical Therapy are trained in the technique, but it is more of a specialty and thus not generally offered.

Structural programs are implemented for three or four months on average, at a frequency of twice per week at the start. As improvement occurs frequency can diminish, but the program continues until normal function and balance has been restored.

Nerve irritation

A major cause of nerve irritation involves the "tone" or health of your vagus nerve, a major cranial nerve affecting most organs in your body. The vagus nerve is known as the "wandering nerve" because it starts in your brain, travels through your neck, alongside your carotid artery and jugular veins, and continues its journey into your chest, abdomen and down to your colon. On its journey it sends information throughout your body, touching major organs including your heart, lungs, and abdomen.

Low "tone" or a non-optimally functioning vagus nerve is associated with inflammation, depression, a poor ability to deal with stress and poor emotional regulation. Healthy vagus nerve function, on the other hand, is associated with the opposite symptoms: positive emotional balance, decreased inflammation, normal heart rate, normal blood pressure and healthy digestion.

The vagus nerve and its function explains how the function of your stomach and digestive tract can be linked to your stress level. It is the job of the vagus nerve to interconnect all these parts of your body.

Considering the "tone" or health of the vagus nerve is connected to inflammatory levels, stress levels, heart rate and a variety of disease states (including heart disease, autoimmune diseases such as rheumatoid arthritis, Alzheimer's, Crohn's, M.S., and cluster headaches, to name a few), how do you ensure its health and proper function?

A healthy vagus nerve releases a neurotransmitter (acetylcholine), linked to the part of your nervous system called the parasympathetic nervous system. The parasympathetic nervous system is tied to your ability to rest, digest, and relax. Acetylcholine is like nature's tranquilizer: clearly something you are not producing in adequate amounts when you have anxiety, feel stressed, or have trouble sleeping.

When your parasympathetic nervous system is not engaged, your sympathetic (fight or flight) nervous system takes over. In the description of the sympathetic nervous system you will likely see yourself if you suffer from anxiety. The sympathetic (fight or flight) nervous system raises your heart rate, increases your anxiety, and raises your blood pressure, to name a few associated symptoms.

Interestingly, one way to increase your production of acetylcholine and "turn on" your parasympathetic nervous system is to breathe deeply from your belly. Slow, deep belly or diaphragmatic breathing is a great tool. It turns out that your vagal "tone" is closely tied into such deep breathing.

If you have Hiatal Hernia Syndrome and your diaphragm is elevated or spasmed, you are unable to perform this activity, leaving you "stuck" in a sympathetic environment. It is this state that must be addressed to provide you the relief you deserve.

If nerve irritation is present, it can affect the function of your diaphragm and related structures. Chiropractic care is one tool that normalizes the function of nerves in your body.

Your diaphragm is a muscle, and like all muscles, it is controlled by nerve impulses. If these nerve impulses are diminished in capacity or intensity, then the diaphragm can become too lax, allowing the stomach to move up through the opening or sphincter.

A chiropractic adjustment removes the misalignments in the spine that have been causing the diminished and improper nerve flow. The treatment restores nerve function and essentially "wakes up" the muscles in the diaphragm.

There is a nerve that travels to your diaphragm which originates in your lower neck; it is called the phrenic nerve. If you notice tightness, stiffness or pain in your neck, the phrenic nerve could be irritated.

Spinal Alignment

The upper part of the lumbar spine (your low back) can subluxate, or move out of position, affecting normal function of the diaphragm. In a study of two hundred cases of Hiatal Hernia

Syndrome[15], researcher Edmunds found spinal deformity of the lumbar in sixty percent of the patients.

Often the pelvis is misaligned as well, contributing to the lumbar spine misalignment. The lower back and pelvis are more of a secondary area when it comes to Hiatal Hernia Syndrome, but if the problem is persisting it is worth investigating with the help of a Doctor of Chiropractic.

The psoas muscles

The psoas (pronounced SO-az) muscles are a common contributor to Hiatal Hernia Syndrome and we will spend some time discussing them. The psoas are frequently reactive with the diaphragm and are a common cause of diaphragmatic dysfunction.

The psoas muscles may be the most important muscles in your body. Structurally they are the deepest muscles in your core. They begin at your spine in your lower back and pelvis and end at your inner thigh bones, the femurs.

Why are they so important?

They are major postural muscles, and the only muscles that connect your spine to your legs. If you are standing, they stabilize your spine, maintaining the normal position of your lower and middle back.

They are such an essential muscle group that if it they were not functioning properly you would not even be able to get out of bed in the morning. Whether you run, bike, dance, practice yoga or

---

15   Edmunds, V. *"Hiatus hernia – a clinical study of 200 cases"*, QJ Med, Vol 26 No 104 (Oct '57)

just sit on your couch, your psoas muscles are involved. They act as the connector between your torso and your legs, affecting your posture and the stability of your spine.

The action of your psoas muscles is as follows: when they contract, it brings your knee in towards your stomach. If you spend a lot of time sitting, your psoas are likely tight because the sitting position shortens the muscles.

How do the psoas play into Hiatal Hernia Syndrome?

The psoas muscles support your internal organs in a unique way. They work like a pump, moving blood and lymph in and out of your cells.

The connection to your diaphragm is rather fascinating. The diaphragm has two tendons (crura) that extend down, connecting to your spine alongside the psoas muscles. One of the ligaments wraps around the top of each of your psoas muscles.

Your diaphragm and psoas muscles are connected through a specialized connective tissue called fascia that also connects to other hip muscles. It is this connection that ties your psoas muscles to your diaphragm, connecting your ability to walk to how you breathe.

Due to this connection between your psoas and your diaphragm, an in-depth examination of your psoas is part of our hiatal hernia structural examination.

We evaluate for the following:

- Leg length discrepancy. You can have involvement of one psoas muscle more than the other, resulting in differing leg length.

- Knee and low back pain. These can be caused from psoas imbalance, which essentially locks your femur (thigh bone) into your hip socket such that normal rotation cannot occur. This in turn causes abnormal torque on your lower back and knee.

- Postural problems. If the psoas is tight it can pull your pelvis out of position, creating a "duck butt". If it is weak, the reverse occurs, and you have a "flat butt". Neither is normal and can cause low back or hip pain and injury.

- Difficulty moving your bowels. It may seem odd that a muscle imbalance could affect your colon, but it is true. A large group of nerves and blood vessels pass around and through the psoas muscle. Tightness of the muscle can affect both flood flow and nerve impulses, contributing to constipation.

- Menstrual cramps. In the same fashion as the psoas can affect bowel function, imbalance can affect reproductive organs, particularly the uterus, aggravating menstrual cramps.

- Chest breathing. A tight psoas muscle can move your ribcage forward, causing shallow chest breathing. This not only delivers less oxygen, but the chest breathing over-utilizes your trapezoids and neck muscles, often creating tension in these areas.

- Feeling exhausted. As you take deep diaphragmatic breaths, your psoas muscles "massage" your kidneys and adrenal glands, stimulating circulation. Psoas tension restricts this motion and adrenal fatigue (or exhaustion) can result. It is fascinating that there exists a connection between your psoas muscle and the fight or flight response of your nervous system. It is believed that when you are under stress, suffering anxiety or even excited, your psoas muscle contracts. Stress that is prolonged can cause a long-term contraction and shortening of your psoas, in much the same way that prolonged sitting does.

In summary, this one muscle not only affects your diaphragm function, but your ability to walk, breathe and how you will respond to stress. It is truly fascinating and hopefully it makes sense to you why our evaluation always includes an in-depth assessment of psoas function.

Somato-visceral response

The connection between the structural aspects of your body and how they affect the functioning of your organs is known as the somato-visceral response. Soma means body; viscera means organs.

Understanding this explains why "physical care" of the body can affect organ function and vice versa. It will now make sense why your chronic stomach inflammation can cause irritation to the nerves that control it, located in the mid-back of your spine. The result can be middle back pain and muscle tension.

The chiropractic pull-down technique

There is a technique taught to some Doctors of Chiropractic during their training. It does not appear to be standard in all curricula, and like anything, it takes practice to excel at it.

It has been commonly called a "pull-down" technique because that is what is felt by the patient, but let us discuss what it actually does.

When done correctly, this non-invasive technique acts as a

mechanical release between the tissues that line your abdominal cavity. It is more properly called "mechanical fascial release of the abdominal peritoneum tissue," but we can agree that is a mouthful!

This technique can not only provide great relief from discomfort, it can also free up your ability to take a deep breath.

We have had some patients weep from the relief they experience when they are able to take their first deep breath in a long time.

Two things to know about this technique:

1. The Doctor of Chiropractic needs to be well trained and have extensive experience to perform it correctly.

2. It is PART your treatment program, not the full treatment. We mention this because we have had patients receive such good relief in their breathing, that they confuse the temporary relief for full treatment.

We are attempting complete correction of your problem, not temporary relief. Don't get me wrong; the relief is great. We perform this technique often on those who suffer. But the end goal is to correct the problem at its root, eliminating the necessity of this technique in the future.

That is not to say the occasional rushed meal or overeating will not be assisted by this technique – it will. But again, the goal is full resolution of your hiatal hernia.

In summary

We have treated unresolved Hiatal Hernia Syndrome with a combination of the above methods for many years. Our successful treatment protocol for a hiatal hernia is a perfect example of how Functional Medicine, Chiropractic and Physical Therapy can work together for the patient's greater good.

The multiple specialties so necessary for the successful treatment of Hiatal Hernia Syndrome epitomizes why Root Cause Medical Clinic is made up of the team of clinicians it is.

Not only does successful treatment begin with a correct diagnosis (often despite a negative traditional test), it also requires understanding the various treatment modalities required to truly fix the problem. It may, and frequently does, involve the teamwork of medical doctors, Functional Medicine doctors, Doctors of Chiropractic, and Doctors of Physical Therapy.

Is Hiatal Hernia Syndrome ever fixed "for good"?

We certainly hear this question often and it is a good one.

The answer is yes, no, and it depends. Let me elaborate.

We have discussed the wide variety of symptoms associated with Hiatal Hernia Syndrome. We have also discussed an equally long list of causes. Treatment varies depending on the cause, of course.

Can the problem be completely fixed? Yes, we have certainly seen that in many cases.

When does it not "stay fixed"? If you stop doing the successful actions that fixed the problem, the syndrome can return.

We see it frequently. Patients are delighted to have their problem resolved. They continue to do the right actions for a while, be it dietary change, keeping their weight in check, exercising, etc.

Then time passes. They "forget" about how bad they felt earlier. They "cheat" a bit on their diet and notice no negative effects. They "cheat" more, and more, and pretty soon they are back to their old, unhealthy habits.

"Suddenly" (although it is not truly sudden) they are not feeling well anymore. Depending on their circumstances, they might reach for the antacids again. Or wonder if they are suddenly developing anxiety for some other reason.

We could give you a hundred different examples of this.

Sometimes, the patient is maintaining what they have been told to do, but life throws a curve ball at them. A woman has a baby, and it is a big baby that weakens her abdominal muscles and forces her diaphragm to elevate. An individual has a surgery, and the surgery throws their digestive tract out of balance, resulting in acid reflux or constipation.

There are many circumstances that could cause the syndrome to recur.

The great news is that your body loves to heal. The best action to take is to reach out to your clinician who fixed the problem in the first place and have him or her find out what is creating the current symptoms.

There is no reason your problem cannot again be resolved.

CHAPTER 12

HOME REMEDIES AND HOME TESTS

Hiatal Hernia Syndrome is very common, and its incidence is increasing as our American diet continues to worsen and obesity levels rise, all while a lack of exercise and sedentary lifestyle become more common.

In this chapter we cover some home tests and remedies that may provide for you some temporary relief.

The home remedies are not treatment, because effective treatment would include resolution.

They also do not obviate the need for you to contact your doctor to ensure you do not have a condition that requires medical treatment.

Why then do we include a chapter on "home remedies" that provide only temporary relief, if any? We will tell you. Nothing makes us sadder than to "meet" someone (in person or over long distance) whom we know we can help, but we are unable to do so.

It may be someone who lives in an area of the country where their local doctor is providing no help, but they are unable, financially, to receive our help.

Or it may be someone living outside the U.S. and unable to move forward with even remote telemedicine care.

There are many such reasons that preclude us from providing the care they need, but the bottom line is that it is frustrating for both of us.

Knowledge is power and some of the data in this chapter may provide some meaningful relief until you can find the comprehensive help you need. It is my hope that this book will "open the eyes" of not just patients but practitioners alike. With such increased awareness will come increased availability for effective treatment, something that is presently sadly lacking.

Home Tests

Let us begin with two home tests to assess your breathing capacity. As you know, Hiatal Hernia Syndrome tends to cause malfunction of the diaphragm, compromising your ability to breath normally. These tests can be performed on your own or with someone else assisting you; there is no liability to performing them.

Ventilation Test

An interesting and easy test to assess sufficiency of ventilation is to take a lit match, place it six inches from a person's wide-open mouth and see if they can blow out the match without pursing their lips.

The test is designed to check expiration sufficiency with the mouth wide open. The examiner ensures he or she is holding the match at the proper level to meet the force of air coming from the patient's open mouth.

Inability to complete the test successfully is associated with diaphragmatic weakness or reduced thoracic cage mobility (assuming there is no lung disease present).

Home diagnosis of proper diaphragmatic expansion

The easiest way to tell if you or someone you know has poor diaphragm motion is to place your fingers on the solar plexus, just below the tip of the breastbone.

While keeping your fingers there, take a deep breath.

You should feel the solar plexus expand and move outward.

If there is no movement at the solar plexus and instead the person must lift their chest and shoulders to take a deep breath, then your diaphragm is not moving correctly, and hiatal hernia may be a cause.

You should be able to take a deep abdominal breath without lifting your shoulders.

Home Remedies

There are several home remedies to be found online. Understand: none of them is a cure, but we are citing them here as they may provide you some temporary relief.

Here at Root Cause Medical Clinics we are focused on correction and repair, not temporary "band-aids", but if you try any of the below and gain some relief, there is certainly no harm, as long as you understand that it is temporary and that your focus should be true resolution of the entire syndrome, as much as it is possible.

If we seem to be "beating a dead horse" about the concept of relief vs. correction, it is simply because we live in a completely relief-oriented health care model, one that we feel does us a grave injustice. Correction is at hand, typically drug-free, and it opens the door for a long and healthy life.

The Warm Water Technique

This technique is to be done first thing in the morning on an empty stomach. It is designed to assist in breaking the spasm between the stomach and diaphragm.

Please note, we are not the authors of this procedure.

1. While still in bed, drink a glass of slightly warm water. This should relax the stomach muscles and diaphragm and create some weight in your stomach from the water.

2. Once you have drunk the water, stand up and lift your arms straight out from your sides at chest level.

3. With your shoulders back, bend your arms at your elbows so your hands touch your chest. (This position is designed to open the opening between your stomach and esophagus while stretching your diaphragm.)

4. Maintaining this position, stand on your toes and drop down heavily on to your heels. Repeat this maneuver a few times. The goal is that the weight of the water in your stomach will help to pull it down, breaking the spasm between it and your diaphragm.

5. The final step is to raise your arms overhead and pant with your mouth open several times, for about fifteen seconds total. The panting is designed to tighten the diaphragm and close the esophageal sphincter, or opening, now that your stomach is in a lower, more normal position.

Note: If this feels uncomfortable at any point, simply stop. This maneuver offers temporary relief for some, but not for everyone. If it does not aggravate you, it cannot hurt to try it.

Self-Massage Technique

In my experience, patients frequently intuit this technique to relieve their discomfort. Again, this is for temporary relief; if it provides some abatement of symptoms, it certainly cannot hurt if done gently.

1. Lie on your back and relax. (Ensure you have an empty stomach.)

2. Place your fingers just below your rib cage.

3. Apply a downward pressure and slowly move your hands from just below your ribs, down towards your belly button. You can massage on the right, left and midline, wherever you are feeling most uncomfortable.

4. Continue the massage for about five minutes.

Note: Do not perform the massage on a full stomach. Wait at least thirty to forty-five minutes or more after eating before performing this technique. If this helps you relax and feel better, perform the massage twice per day.

Baking Soda Relief

Baking soda is a natural antacid and can provide relief from heartburn rather quickly.

For relief, add ½ teaspoon to a glass of warm water and drink immediately.

Note: Do not utilize it if you have high blood pressure. A side effect of baking soda is that it can cause salt retention, thereby aggravating a high blood pressure condition.

You can repeat this as needed but it is important to not utilize it excessively, and only away from meals. Baking soda can compromise your digestion, something that is already a problem if you have Hiatal Hernia Syndrome.

Baking Soda Low Acid Test

This test is used to help you determine if your stomach acid is diminished.

Mix ¼ teaspoon baking soda in 4-6 ounces of cold water first thing in morning before eating or drinking anything.

Drink the solution.

Time how long it takes you to burp or belch. If you have not burped nor belched within five minutes, this is a sign of low stomach acid production.

Apple Cider Vinegar for Acid Reflux

The anecdotal evidence for treating acid reflux with apple cider vinegar (ACV) is robust, the scientific evidence less so. Many cite there is no scientific research, but we did find a study performed by a graduate student from Arizona State University.

It is not peer-reviewed, but it is a randomized, placebo-controlled, double-blind, cross-over research study. It was a thesis paper, therefore obtaining a master's degree was predicated on a well-done study titled *"Is Apple Cider Vinegar Effective for Reducing Heartburn Symptoms Related to Gastroesophageal Reflux Disease?"* by Zoe Yeh[16].

The research evaluated heartburn after eating chili four ways:

1. Chili alone, no antacid or apple cider vinegar (ACV)
2. Chili with an antacid taken after a meal
3. Chili that had organic apple cider vinegar added to it
4. Drinking diluted organic apple cider vinegar after the chili meal.

---

16   *"Is Apple Cider Vinegar Effective for Reducing Heartburn Symptoms Related to Gastroesophageal Reflux Disease?"* by Zoe Yeh

Those taking the ACV did as well as those who took antacids, as regards heartburn symptoms. There was no significant difference among each type of treatment.

The author of the study felt that a large study needed to be performed, but despite the small size, it certainly was a well-designed study that showed ACV performing on par with antacids.

Most treatments recommend between a teaspoon and a tablespoon of organic apple cider vinegar diluted into a glass of water. It can be taken before or after the meal for acid reflux symptoms.

There are multiple theories as to why it works. It has been suggested that ACV helps to balance the stomach's pH levels, neutralizing excess acid.

Others suggest that acid reflux can be the result of too little stomach acid (not too much) and ACV adds the needed additional acid into the stomach.

Still others point to the acetic acid contained in ACV as having anti-microbial benefits. This would improve your ability to fight against any inhospitable bacteria present that may be contributing to reflux.

If you really want to give ACV a try, know there are also pill forms available that can bypass the unpleasant taste of drinking the vinegar. Beyond taste, the pill will not "get to work" until it arrives in your stomach, which will also decrease any irritation of an inflamed esophagus, which the liquid can cause.

Chewing Gum

A small study had participants chew sugar-free gum for thirty minutes after lunch or dinner, and it appeared to reduce acid levels in the esophagus (acid reflux). Consider trying this, but it is likely best to avoid mint flavors as these have been found to exacerbate acid reflux in some.

Also, avoid artificial sweeteners. Consider xylitol, which is also protective of your teeth.

Not everyone is bothered by peppermint or spearmint but do your trial with another flavor first and if you meet with success, then try a mint flavor to see if there is a difference.

There is no harm in trying gum, provided you avoid dangerous artificial sweeteners and sugar-containing gum.

Aloe Vera Juice

When you think of aloe vera, you likely think of its ability to reduce the effects of sunburn. This is due to its anti-inflammatory properties.

Beyond its topical use, it appears to have internal benefits as well.

There are pros and cons of using aloe vera, so please read this entire section before trying it.

A 2015 study was published in the *Journal of Chinese Medicine,* titled *"Efficacy and Safety of Aloe Vera Syrup for the Treatment of Gastroesophageal Reflux Disease: A Pilot Randomized Positive-Controlled Trial.*[17]*"*

---

17   National Library of Medicine, PubMed.gov *"Efficacy and safety of Aloe vera syrup for the treatment of gastroesophageal reflux disease: a pilot randomized positive-*

Utilizing decolorized and purified aloe vera juice, the researchers found it may be a safe and effective treatment for reducing reflux symptoms.

The aloe vera juice effectively reduced the symptoms of acid reflux, as did certain traditional medications, all without any reported side effects. For some participants, the aloe vera juice was more effective than traditional medication.

The conclusion was that the aloe vera juice acted as both an anti-inflammatory agent and an acid reducer.

Begin with a dose of one to two tablespoons to see how you tolerate it.

That is the good news, but there are important things to consider before you jump on the aloe vera juice bandwagon.

- Decolorized and purified aloe vera juice from a trusted source is required. This is the type of aloe vera best tolerated, with minimal side effects.

- Aloe vera juice can cause diarrhea in some individuals; this is typically the non-decolorized type, which contains a strong laxative and potential intestinal irritant (anthraquinone). This is an example of why quality is so important when it comes to aloe vera.

- If you have diabetes, know that aloe vera can amplify the effects of diabetes medication. This could result in your blood sugar levels going too low. Therefore, it is important to discuss this with your doctor before starting.

- Drinking aloe vera juice may induce miscarriage.

---

controlled trial"

- Avoid aloe vera juice if you are taking diuretics or laxatives.

Hopefully, this chapter has provided you with some palliative, drug-free measures that you can take while looking for a clinician who can help remedy your Hiatal Hernia Syndrome.

CHAPTER 13

CAUTIONS – KNOWING WHEN TO SEEK EMERGENCY MEDICAL HELP

I n this book we have reviewed the long list of potential symptoms associated with Hiatal Hernia Syndrome (HHS). These symptoms can be miserable, painful, and frightening, not to mention anxiety-provoking.

If you have been to the E.R. or Urgent Care on numerous occasions in the past, only to be told "you are fine," you are not alone. It is extremely common for me to hear that from my patients.

After a while, you start to put up with your symptoms, regardless of how miserable you feel, because you see no point in hearing the same diagnosis of: "You are fine," or "You have acid reflux, here is a pill," or "You are having a panic attack, here is a mind-altering medication".

It is very understandable why you would not want repeat visits when you are receiving no help.

We do want to make the distinction here of symptoms that do warrant seeking out emergency care or an urgent call to your doctor.

These severe symptoms include the following:

- Severe chest pain – the pain is intense, and you feel like you may be having a heart attack
- Sudden nausea and vomiting, especially if you are vomiting any blood
- Great difficulty breathing – feeling like you are choking or wheezing and are getting short of air
- Severe constipation or severe abdominal bloating or gas
- Your voice gets extremely hoarse.

If you or a loved one are experiencing any of the above it is best to be safe and seek out medical help to ensure there is nothing requiring emergency intervention.

CHAPTER 14

PATIENT SUCCESS STORIES

What follows are success stories our patients have chosen to share about their journey to improved health after suffering Hiatal Hernia Syndrome.

If you would like to watch some video testimonials, visit our website at *www.RootCauseMedicalClinics.com*.

> *"I started going to Root Cause Medical Clinic earlier this year. I'm in my early thirties and had a lot of stress and changes in my life for more than a year and a half leading up to the consultation visit.*
>
> *"My immunity had taken a nosedive and I racked up a list of ailments — a couple had been more long term, but not serious by conventional standards. I wanted to finally get things under control and find out why I wasn't getting better.*

"I did visit several conventional medical doctors who were well-intentioned, but mostly unhelpful.

"I also did some research and found that I had symptoms of a hiatal hernia.

"After my evaluation, which confirmed hiatal hernia syndrome, I started a combined physical therapy and chiropractic program. Dr. Rupa, Dr. Sterling and the PT team are awesome to work with and they've given me a lot of relief.

"On the internal medicine side of the clinic, the supplements and dietary and lifestyle changes Dr. Rick prescribed are also making a big difference with my digestion.

"I've seen improvements, and I did a follow-up lab test that confirmed one of the significant treatments worked.

"I was also recently tested for mold toxicity and have started the protocol for that.

"I'll definitely continue my treatments with the clinic as I still have a ways to go, but I am very pleased with my results so far.

"They work with my health savings account, which has been so helpful. Getting treatment is an investment. The front desk team is really accommodating, thoughtful and professional!

"I would recommend!"

- Abigail B.

❧

"I started seeing the team at Root Cause Medical Clinic about seven weeks ago. I was skeptical simply because it's an alternative medicine practice and I think most people aren't privy to anything beyond traditional medicine.

"However, their team is very attentive and proactive in listening and attending to resolving the underlying issues.

"My main reason for the visit was to find relief from three years of suffering from chest pains, GI issues, headaches and anxiety. I came to find out that all of my symptoms are most likely caused by hiatal hernia, a condition typically misdiagnosed by traditional medicine.

"The staff developed a plan for an elimination diet, in order to help find out if some type of food is creating the symptoms. To be honest, the diet is terrible, especially for the first three weeks as your body is adjusting. However, it does get better.

"Subsequently, I started working with the PT and chiropractor to adjust the alignment of my spine and hip (caused from a motorcycle accident). This might sound odd, but it was explained that since the spine and hip are misplaced it could have led to the hiatal hernia, and other symptoms associated.

"Long story short, after seven weeks I'm feeling much better. All the chest pains and GI issues have been significantly reduced. I am able to eat a lot of different foods now that were causing me trouble before.

"Overall, after suffering for three years, I am happy with Root Cause Medical Clinic and owe them credit for helping me out."

-Rob B.

"I've been seeing alternative specialists for decades, yet no one has provided such a comprehensive, caring program as the doctors and staff at Root Cause Medical Clinic.

"From the lovely, uber-efficient ladies at the front desk, to the

knowledgeable experts in the Physical Therapy department, this facility is worth the high price tag, because they really care about healing the ailments that burden us, and they are determined to get results.

"I've been seeing these doctors and specialists regularly for over four months, initially for chronic digestive discomfort, then for other problems as well.

"They have diminished or completely eliminated my symptoms of hiatal hernia, back pain, and muscle tightness; helped to improve my postural faults; balanced my digestive problems; provided vast information and counsel on diet and nutritional improvements, and given wise, professional advice on my future health maintenance.

"Co-founder Dr. Vikki Petersen served as my introduction to the clinic, having seen her fascinating lecture on the grim reality of Gluten Intolerance, which persuaded me to trust her approach.

"Many thanks to Dr. Rick Petersen for his investigative, hard-science testing for the resolution of my digestive problems. The numerous lab tests proved to be beneficial in isolating several hidden problems that needed to be addressed, in order for my intestinal tract to be healed – or at least to be set in the right direction for a complete healing.

"Other practitioners in the past have fallen short in their diagnoses.

"Dr. Haglund is a smart MD who embraces a more holistic viewpoint towards health, and I'm grateful for her collaborative advice, as well.

"Rachel, the Registered Dietitian, is an encyclopedia of nutritional information, keeping up to date on the best food products and trends in the whole foods industry.

"Dr. Sterling Petersen is a young, efficient and precise chiropractor with a tableside manner that is hipster-cool and friendly. His well-dressed appearance, like his father/mentor Dr. Rick, adds a professional, upscale touch to this clinic, which one might expect in the Saratoga neighborhood.

"Dr. Rupa is an experienced and trustworthy doctor of physical therapy and director of her department, who keeps the PT team running efficiently, aided by her staff of superb associates.

"Returning to the front-of-the-house staff, this team are the friendliest and most efficient of any medical office that I've ever encountered. And I've encountered many.

"After the months I've spent in their care, I'm getting well, gradually but certainly, because of the combined efforts of this excellent team, who also reinforce the necessity of me doing my homework on myself, and not being dependent on them forever.

"I highly recommend their philosophy and their practice."

- Bianca C.

∽

"Things first started to go wrong earlier this year, back in January. I started to feel like I couldn't breathe and had shortness of breath. I ended up going to the ER with really high blood pressure and overall, just wasn't feeling good.

"I went to the ER a bunch of times throughout the year. I had high blood pressure, shortness of breath, chest pain, and even high cholesterol. None of the doctors could figure out what was wrong with me. I took a lot of tests to try to figure it out and finally they found the hiatal hernia on an angiogram (heart exam) by accident.

"But the hiatal hernia was dismissed as nothing. So, after doing a whole bunch of tests, seeing a bunch of specialists, and going to the ERs ten times, I still had no answers.

"The hiatal hernia was confirmed on an endoscopy and the doctor gave me an antacid for four weeks. I saw no benefit and was then told to wait eight weeks. When that didn't work, I was told to take a stronger drug and wait another eight weeks.

"They kept doubling my medication and I felt no better. I started to realize there really is no treatment. There really was no understanding of my problem.

"When I went back to my PCP complaining, I was told that hiatal hernia doesn't cause shortness of breath or, in fact, any of the symptoms I had. I was told that my problem was anxiety and I needed to go see a psychologist or a psychiatrist. I was quickly prescribed an antidepressant.

"I took every pill they told me to take and I wasn't getting better.

"You get to the point that you realize it's time to try something different. My wife and I began surfing the internet and looking for answers.

"We came across the video by Dr. Vikki Petersen and the Root Cause Medical Clinic. What Dr Vikki explained about hiatal hernia syndrome matched pretty much everything that was going on with me. I left a comment describing my symptoms on the YouTube video. I was offered a free consultation, so I called.

"Everything was immediate; I got an immediate response. Since I was so severe, having suffered the past eleven months, the clinic got me in right away and understood what was going on.

"The doctors here at Root Cause educated me about my condition. The doctors taught me specifically what was going on with my nerves and with my diaphragm. Specific lab tests were done to check what might be causing it.

"The team are working with me to fix it, to make me better again. I like that I'm also being educated on how I can help myself with my diet, physical therapy exercises at home and lifestyle changes.

"This is so different from the approach of a regular, traditional doctor, who comes from a position of authority, that 'You have anxiety; take this pill' and there is no disputing it. And if you keep feeling bad, it's only because of your anxiety, so take an even stronger dose until eventually, you know, you're just going to be so 'out of it' from all the drugs they're giving you. It's not a good way to treat people; it doesn't make sense to me at all.

"When I came here to Root Cause it all made sense...I realized the doctors of Root Cause do know what's going on with me and how to fix it. This made me feel a lot better.

"I'm very appreciative to everyone here. My symptoms were having a terrible impact on my life. I had shortness of breath, headaches, and it was very difficult for me to think, speak or move around. I was very fatigued. It ended up keeping me out of work for close to a year.

"I work in a security job that requires me to be mentally and physically alert. I was no longer capable of doing my job, which could put lives at risk. I had severe brain fog, a very difficult time trying to find the right words, and low comprehension and situational awareness.

"Regarding my treatment here, changing my diet improved my symptoms right away. It helped me big time. Plus, the education and guidance on what I can and cannot eat was super helpful. The chiropractic and physical therapy treatments, adjusting my diaphragm and the nerves of my neck and back are really *making a difference also. The treatment is very precise, and I can tell the doctors know exactly what they're doing.*

"My breathing is better and so is my brain fog. I'm comprehending better and don't feel so confused. My acid reflux is improving also. I feel like all the treatments – diet, nutrition and physical – are all working together.

"I feel like you guys are my super team and you have my back. And that feels really good because I've been suffering with this for a very long time.

"I'm sharing this because I know there are others out there suffering and I hope my story and sharing what the team here can do will help others.

"If you want to go see a team of doctors with outstanding expertise, knowledge, and experience, you should visit the doctors at Root Cause Medical Clinic. I drove nine hours to get here because I believe health should be your number one priority.

"Thank you for helping me to be a better version of myself."

- Michael F.

෯

"I can't say enough good things about Root Cause! Everything that you need to accomplish, all of your wellness goals is under one roof, whether it's chiropractic, physical therapy, nutrition or functional medicine.

"All of the doctors and staff are incredibly knowledgeable and friendly, and genuinely interested in seeing their patients heal. I came to the clinic to be treated for a hiatal hernia, which was making me feel miserable, and greatly affecting my quality of life.

"I am now on a treatment plan put together by the wonderful doctors at the clinic, that is yielding me great results! I highly recommend Root Cause, especially if you have digestive issues and/or a hiatal hernia. Thank you, Root Cause, for everything. I am a fan for life!"

– D.W.

෴

"I'm writing my story in the hope it will help others!

"A couple of years ago I started developing uncomfortable symptoms after eating. I would have shortness of breath and slight chest pain and pressure.

"I got it checked out by my traditional medical doctor and he concluded it was just acid reflux. After taking acid reflux medicine for a couple of months, things only got worse. I had more chest pain, could hardly eat anything without getting short of breath and feeling very full and bloated (yes, even a salad created these symptoms).

"After seeing no results, I got a second opinion from a gastroenterologist. They performed an upper endoscopy and told me that I did not have any signs of acid reflux, but I did have a slight hiatal hernia. They told me this hernia was not causing any of my symptoms. They thought I had a 'sensitive nerve' in my esophagus and was suffering from anxiety, so they prescribed me anti-depressants.

"I was very skeptical of taking these pills as I have never thought that I was an anxious person at all. After three to four months of taking these pills I started to develop more symptoms in addition to the original ones I had started with. Now I had

heart palpitations, dizziness, and numbness in my feet. All these symptoms occurred after eating meals.

"One day I ate some fried food and thirty minutes later I had severe shortness of breath, dizziness, chest pain, heart palpitations, and numbness in my limbs. I thought I was having a heart attack. I ended up going to the ER and they did multiple tests. After the tests all came back fine, they said that it was just a panic attack and gave me different anti-depressants to take.

"Nothing got better so I started Googling and researching and came across Root Cause Medical Clinic's website. All the symptoms they described on their website about hiatal hernia syndrome fit me 'to a T' so I decided to give them a call.

"My life changed forever!

"My health has improved tremendously under their care. They ran multiple tests and figured out that I had an H. pylori infection (bacterial infection in the stomach), vitamin deficiencies, and a gluten sensitivity. I had looked into possible gluten intolerance before and tried to eliminate it from my diet, but did not know that you had to take certain steps, like the elimination diet, to see real results from eliminating gluten or any other foods.

"I got treated for the infection and vitamin deficiencies with supplements and probiotics. They were great at not giving too many supplements as some other doctors tend to do. I only had to take three! I was also put on the elimination diet as I mentioned before.

"After about five weeks on the elimination diet I noticed a tremendous difference! My symptoms started to slowly go away, and I was able to do more activities again. I developed so much more energy and my mood improved tremendously. I had no

idea that gluten and vitamin deficiencies could be causing so much havoc on my body!

"My experience at Root Cause Medical Clinic has been amazing. All the doctors have been so helpful and knowledgeable. Unlike traditional doctors, they get to the very root of the issue and do whatever it takes to figure out what is really causing your symptoms, instead of masking them with drugs.

"Rachel, the registered dietitian, is so incredibly knowledgeable and has an answer to every single question about your diet. She is a walking dictionary for nutrition; I found her to be an incredible resource!!

"None of the doctors pushed a bunch of supplements on me and I appreciated it so much.

"I would 100% recommend Root Cause Medical Clinic to anyone that I meet. The doctors are way ahead of the game when it comes to medicine. I hope one day that this sort of treatment is common in every doctor's office.

"I want so badly to spread the word of the great things that Root Cause Medical Clinic does for people, so people suffering like I was can find great relief. The money spent and time spent for visits are so worth it!

"Your health is everything!"

- Maggie B.

❧

"I can't say enough good things about Root Cause! Everything that you need to accomplish, all of your wellness goals is under

one roof, whether it's chiropractic, physical therapy, nutrition or functional medicine.

"All of the doctors and staff are incredibly knowledgeable and friendly, and genuinely interested in seeing their patients heal. I came to the clinic to be treated for a hiatal hernia, which was making me feel miserable, and greatly affecting my quality of life.

"I am now on a treatment plan put together by the wonderful doctors at the clinic, that is yielding me great results! I highly recommend Root Cause, especially if you have digestive issues and/or a hiatal hernia. Thank you, Root Cause, for everything. I am a fan for life!"

– Diana W.

CHAPTER 15

RECIPES

In this chapter Dr Vikki offers you a wide array of healthy recipes for breakfast, snacking, entrees, and desserts.

If you are turning to this chapter before you have read CHAPTER 8: DOS AND DON'TS, and CHAPTER 11: TREATMENT, please go back and read those. The DOS AND DON'TS will be helpful in your understanding of certain foods that can aggravate your acid reflux. The TREATMENT chapter will emphasize the power of food and importance of avoiding food sensitivities.

There are many aspects to successful treatment of Hiatal Hernia Syndrome, but a "must" for everyone is to identify and avoid food sensitivities. There are few things you can state as "always true," but when it comes to patients with Hiatal Hernia Syndrome, we do not feel we are overstating it to say there is almost always a food sensitivity present.

It is for that reason I thought it would be helpful to share recipes that avoid the most common food sensitivities we encounter with our patients. All the recipes in this chapter are free of gluten, dairy, and sugar, and are plant-based.

If you are allergic to nuts, please note that nuts are used liberally with many of the desserts, so you will need to adapt with seeds, butters made from sunflower seeds, and flours made from grains rather than almonds.

The recipes are not just low-allergy, but also health-promoting – filled with great nutrition that nourishes you, is anti-inflammatory and immune boosting.

Spicy recipes are not included. We find that when acid reflux is severe, raw onions, peppers, citrus and tomatoes can be aggravating. Cooking the onions and garlic, especially slowly, can make a difference for many, so you can give that a try since the health benefits are profound.

I am Italian and the family joke is that I start every meal sautéing garlic and onions while I decide what I am going to prepare. That is an exaggeration, but I will confess to using them liberally. Do not be concerned if they are bothersome for you even if cooked; I have some solutions. If you have enjoyed them in the past, please know that once you heal you should be able to reintroduce them into your diet.

In the meantime, asofoetida can be your new "best friend" while you need to avoid onions and garlic. Known as "food of the gods," asofoetida is made from fennel. The sap is extracted, and the root is dried to create a vibrant yellow resin which smells like garlic. When used in cooking the aroma substitutes beautifully for onions and garlic.

Small amounts are all that is needed. A ½ teaspoon can be substituted for two cloves of minced garlic or ⅔ cup of minced onion.

It is great when serving guests that are sensitive or for those who wish to avoid onion or garlic breath.

For a more inclusive recipe library, visit my website at: *www.Root-CauseMedicalClinics.com*. There are literally hundreds of recipes, more than I could include here.

RECIPES

Desserts | 321

RECIPES

BREAKFAST

FLUFFY BANANA PANCAKES

Pancakes just scream breakfast, although I know some people who partake for dinner on occasion. There is something special about pancakes that elevates breakfast. It is probably the fact that they are a bit laborious to make or that one usually enjoys them at a restaurant.

Unfortunately, traditional pancakes are loaded with gluten, milk, sugar, and eggs. For those with gluten reactions there really has not been a decent alternative. I have tried some recipes in the past, but they were gluey and far from fluffy or delicious.

But imagine a pancake that isn't just healthy for you but delicious AND easy AND fast! Now we have a winner. All you need to do is throw a few ingredients into your blender and you're ready.

You can top with organic berries of your choice, stevia chocolate chips, bananas, hemp seeds, cinnamon, etc. Also consider throwing some fruit or chocolate chips in the pancake before you flip it.

Let us know the combinations you come up with and how you enjoy these super easy yet healthy pancakes.

Ingredients

1 heaping cup organic gluten-free rolled oats

¼ cup non-dairy, unsweetened organic milk

1 ripe organic banana

1 tablespoon baking powder

1 tablespoon organic apple cider vinegar

1 tablespoon organic maple syrup

1 teaspoon vanilla extract

½ teaspoon organic cinnamon

small amount of organic avocado oil for cooking

Method

- Combine all the ingredients in a blender and blend until smooth.

- Allow the batter to rest for 5 to 10 minutes, giving the oats time to absorb the liquid and to thicken.

- Preheat a pan over medium high heat and add a scant teaspoon of oil. Once hot, pour in about ¼ cup of batter.

- Cook for 1 to 2 minutes or until you can easily slide a spatula underneath.

- Flip, then cook for another 1 to 2 minutes on the second side.

- Repeat until all the batter is used up.

- Add your toppings of choice and enjoy.

(Recipe courtesy of *The Big Man's World*: *https://thebigmansworld.com/*)

POWER OATMEAL BOWL

Dr. Sterling eats this high protein, gluten-free, plant-based oatmeal bowl. You can change it up depending on the season, enjoying the fresh fruits or nuts in season.

You can make it as unique as you want by adding different nuts, spices or sweeteners.

Start your day off right with this protein-packed oatmeal!

Ingredients

1 cup organic gluten-free Bob's Red Mill Steel Cut Oats

2 ½ cups purified water

a pinch of salt

1 heaping tablespoon organic peanut butter or almond butter, measured according to your love for peanut butter or calorie count (Option: cashew butter or sunflower butter.)

1 small handful organic walnuts, cashews, or almonds

1 small handful organic raisins

Optional: Sweeten to taste using 10 drops SweetLeaf stevia or 1 teaspoon organic maple syrup.

¼ cup organic unsweetened vanilla almond milk, gluten-free oat milk or soy milk

¼ teaspoon organic cinnamon

Toppings of your choice! Bananas, blueberries, strawberries, ground flax, pumpkin or sunflower seeds

Method

- Add water, oats and salt to an Instant Pot and set to 3 minutes to cook. (If you don't have an Instant Pot, just follow directions on oats packaging and cook on a stovetop; consider making it the night before to save time in the morning.)

- Place cooked oats in a bowl.

- Stir in peanut butter.

- Add walnuts, raisins, cinnamon, almond milk, and sweetener.

VANILLA CHIA PUDDING WITH A HEALTHY PUNCH

I love pudding and I love eating ingredients that are healthy. Chia pudding is the perfect combination. It's creamy, luscious, a little sweet, plus it's rich in fiber to keep the gut healthy, and it helps reduce blood pressure – not as well as flax does, but I haven't yet created a delicious one hundred percent flax pudding: stand by for that one.

The available omega-3 fatty acids that do come from the flax in this recipe are proven to reduce inflammatory markers in the blood, thereby reducing your risk of heart disease, diabetes, cancer and overweight.

(**Note:** Remember that chia seeds, just like flax, MUST be ground to enjoy any of their benefits.)

Lignans (actually, their precursors) are what you find in chia, flax and other foods such as whole grains, kale, and sesame seeds – although flax seeds win the prize of having the most lignans of all.

A healthy gut flora is required to turn the precursors into actual lignans, which we can then absorb. This is why we focus on the health of the gut flora with our patients. When it's poor, absorption of nutrients is compromised, along with the ability to detoxify.

We think of our liver as our detoxification organ, but in fact our gut flora, with one hundred trillion organisms, represents an even greater detoxification capacity.

Why do we want to eat lignans? They appear to extend life expectancy, especially in regard to cancer. Intake is associated with improved survival among postmenopausal women with breast cancer – a study revealed it cut mortality risk by fifty percent. Is it only good for women? Nope. Lignans help with prostate health as well.

Chia definitely contains healthy fiber; enjoy it in the form of pudding and your gut will thank you. Please let me know how you enjoy it!

Ingredients

½ cup raw organic almonds, walnuts or pecans

1 to 1 ½ cups filtered water (The amount depends on how you thick you like your pudding.)

2 to 4 pitted organic dates, soaked in hot water for at least 20 minutes (The number depends on how sweet you like your pudding.)

½ teaspoon vanilla extract

a pinch of Himalayan sea salt

2 tablespoons organic chia seeds, ground (Option: Substitute ¼ cup cooked organic quinoa for half the chia seeds.)

¾ tablespoon organic flax seeds, ground

½ teaspoon cinnamon, ground

1 to 2 tablespoons organic raisins (Option: Goji berries or any fresh fruit you'd like to top your pudding.)

Method

- Blend the almonds, water, soaked dates, vanilla and salt in a high-speed blender until smooth and creamy. I recommend starting with about ½ to ¾ cup of water at first to ensure all the almonds get blended. Then you can add the rest of the water as needed to get the thickness you desire.

- Using 1 cup of water, it will be the consistency of a thick milk.

- Adding the chia thickens the mixture considerably. If you like your chia pudding more soupy, add more water so that you start with the consistency of a typical almond milk. If you want the pudding more like mousse, start with a thicker milk.

- Pour into a container that you can cover and refrigerate once you add the chia seeds.

- Add the chia seeds and cinnamon to the milk mixture; stir well and refrigerate for at least a couple of hours or overnight. The pudding will thicken up during this time.

- Remove from the refrigerator and top with raisins or fresh fruit as you desire.

- If for some reason you find the pudding is too thick for your liking, it's very easy to place it in the blender with a little extra almond milk or even coconut milk if you have it on hand.

EASY OVERNIGHT OATS

Healthy, easy, and filling!

We are all busy in the morning and sometimes trying to get out the door on time with a healthy breakfast on board can be a challenge. Smoothies are great but they take time. You can make them the night before, but they really are most nutritious within a few hours of making them.

This recipe is delicious, filling, and easy to prepare – the night before! That's the best part. You just grab it and go in the morning because your refrigerator has done all the "work" while you sleep.

If you are avoiding oats you can try organic quinoa flakes instead. Another option is a quick five-minute buckwheat cereal (I like Bob's Red Mill) that you can also make the night before and just add to it the rest of the ingredients listed below.

The nut butter gives you protein, some healthy fat and staying power. You won't get hungry for several hours.

The flax has healthy omega-3s, fiber and anti-cancer phytonutrients – a true superfood.

I really love playing around with it and making it my own. I hope you enjoy this recipe as much as I do! Feel free to add your favorite ingredients and let me know what varieties you come up with.

Serves 1 (It's a small serving; double the recipe if you're hungry!)

Ingredients

½ cup organic gluten-free rolled oats

1 teaspoon organic chia seeds, ground

1 teaspoon organic ground flax seeds (This is the healthier
option compared to chia, so you can try experimenting
with 2 teaspoons of flax and no chia to see how you like
it.)

1 tablespoon almond butter (peanut or cashew butter are also
options)

¾ cup organic non-dairy milk, such as almond, soy, oat or
coconut

1 tablespoon organic cacao nibs (Option: if these are too
intense for you, substitute chopped nuts or raisins.)

A few drops (up to one dropperful) of SweetLeaf stevia, to
taste. (You can also sweeten with a tablespoon of organic
date syrup.)

Optional: Sometimes in the morning I put in fresh berries or
banana and other times I add cinnamon and raisins.

Method

- Add all ingredients to a clean Mason jar. Combine with a
spoon, cover with a lid, and place in the fridge overnight
or for at least a couple hours. It couldn't be easier!

SOFT AND CHEWY OATMEAL BARS

There are many recipes available for oatmeal bars. But there aren't many that are truly healthy, boasting delicious, soft, chewy sweetness without any gluten, dairy or sugar.

Our clever registered dietitian created these lovely, very simple bars with a few easy ingredients. The filling doubles as a delicious jam by the way, so you can consider making extra and enjoying it where you would enjoy your favorite jam or jelly. This one has zero sugar or preservatives but is addictively delicious.

These bars are sure to be a hit and you can feel completely guilt-free enjoying them as a breakfast bar, snack or dessert. Yes, you can make them *à la mode* for special occasions with some coconut or cashew vanilla "ice cream" in case you were wondering!

Let us know how you enjoy them.

Ingredients

- 1 cup organic almond flour
- ½ cup organic coconut sugar or granulated monk fruit sweetener
- ½ cup Miyoko's vegan butter or organic refined coconut oil
- 1 ½ cups organic gluten-free oats
- 1 teaspoon baking powder
- 3 cups organic strawberries, fresh or frozen
- 2 tablespoons organic lemon juice
- 2 tablespoons organic chia seeds

Method

- Preheat oven to 350°F. Line an eight 8×8" baking dish with parchment paper.

- On the stovetop combine lemon juice, strawberries, and chia seeds over low heat in a medium pan.

- Mash the berries to your desired consistency and stir until the lemon juice is absorbed and the mixture has thickened. Put aside to cool.

- In a medium bowl, combine the dry ingredients, then mix in the melted butter or coconut oil.

- Transfer half of the oat mixture to the baking dish and press to form a flat crust.

- Top with the strawberry mixture and even it out.

- Sprinkle the remaining oat mixture over the top of the strawberries.

- Bake for 25 to 30 minutes until golden brown.

- Cool and enjoy!

DR. VIKKI'S GRANOLA

I have always loved granola. My mother used to make it for me as a kid and it continued to be one of my favorite "care packages" in college. (It is easy to send in the mail as there's nothing to melt or get broken.) Of course, in hindsight it was made with gluten-containing oats and brown sugar, and contained sesame seeds that I happen to be allergic to, but I did not know any of that at the time.

Once we became gluten-free it was still difficult, if not impossible, to find "safe" granola due to the gluten contamination of oats. I still remember the day gluten-free oats became available. I was ecstatic – now I could eat granola again. But it turned out many in the family reacted to oats (as many who are gluten sensitive do) and even the gluten-free variety wasn't going to work.

I decided to create my own with a lot of healthy nuts and seeds, no sugar, and no grains. Too many patients did poorly with grains, and I wanted a nice hearty filling snack option that offered satisfaction through healthy fats and protein, but without the sugar spike.

I hope you enjoy this recipe as much as we do. Organic nuts can get expensive so definitely feel free to go heavier on the seeds and lighter on the nuts if that helps. Another option, if you tolerate gluten-free oats and/or quinoa, consider adding a cup of either to further lower cost.

Total cook time is 35 to 40 min (stir once at halfway point).

Ingredients

- 1 cup organic raw almonds
- 2 cups organic raw cashews
- 1 cup organic raw walnuts

¼ cup organic raw Brazil nuts

¼ cup organic raw flax seeds

1 cup organic raw sunflower seeds

1 cup organic raw pumpkin seeds

Optional: 1 cup organic gluten-free rolled oats

½ cup organic coconut oil, refined or unrefined

½ cup honey or granulated monk fruit

2 teaspoon vanilla

¾ cup shredded organic coconut

½ teaspoon Himalayan sea salt sprinkled on top

2 cups organic raisins

Method

- Preheat oven to 275°F.

- Blend the first four ingredients in a food processor, pulsing until chopped into small pieces. Empty bowl of processor and add the rest of the dry ingredients, pulsing to chop but leaving some larger pieces.

- Combine all the dry ingredients together in a large metal or glass bowl.

- Take a small saucepan and over low heat, melt oil and honey. Stir to combine. Remove from heat and stir in vanilla.

- Add the wet ingredients to the nuts and combine thoroughly until all dry ingredients are coated. Put onto large cookie sheet lined with parchment paper and flatten.

- Place into the oven for 35 to 40 minutes. Stir and turn over at half-way point to make sure nothing is getting too dark. When fully cooked, the granola is a golden brown.

- Add the final three ingredients and stir to combine after you have removed the granola from the oven. Flatten and place in refrigerator to firm up.

SMOOTHIES

GREEN BERRY BREAKFAST SMOOTHIE

Breakfast is an important meal, even if you have it later in the morning. When you are striving to eat more plants, a breakfast smoothie is an easy way to consume about three or four servings of the total daily requirement of nine servings.

We have several options for smoothies because we want you to have variety. Variety is necessary not only so you won't get bored, but also to ensure you get a full complement of nutrients. Mixing up the ingredients you use provides the body with different nutrition.

This is the reason we encourage our patients to eat seasonally. Eating fruits and vegetables in season will assist you in getting a full variety of nutrition from your diet.

I hope you enjoy this smoothie. Let me know of any alternative ingredients you use that make for a delicious outcome. Maybe we'll name our next smoothie after you!

Serves 2

Ingredients

- 2 cups organic baby spinach or organic greens of choice (baby kale is a nice option)
- 1 cup frozen mixed organic berries of berries of choice (raspberries or blueberries add great flavor)

1 organic banana

½ cup of unsweetened organic soy or almond milk, or other
plant-based milk of choice. (You can add more milk if
you like your smoothie thinner. If you like it thicker and
colder, consider adding some ice.)

If you don't have plant-based milk on hand you
can replace it with ½ cup of filtered water and ½ cup of
organic nuts of your choice. Cashews are probably your
best choice because they are a little sweet and will provide
the creamiest texture. Put the nuts in the blender last and
blend until you no longer "hear" them banging around in
the blender.

Optional: ⅛ to ¼ teaspoon of ground cardamom or
cinnamon

Method

- Place plant-based milk, greens of choice, berries and
banana in a high-speed blender on the lowest setting,
advancing up to the highest speed until everything is fully
blended.

- Sprinkle cinnamon on top if desired.

YUMMY, CREAMY HIGH PROTEIN SMOOTHIE

The most common question I get asked when discussing a whole food plant-based diet is, "Where do I get my protein?"

It's a legitimate question: as Americans, the idea that "protein = animal" is ingrained.

Nothing could be farther from the truth, especially if you want to be healthy. There is no comparison between the health benefits provided from plant-based protein vs animal-based protein. Plant-based proteins are anti-cancer, anti-inflammatory and have the added benefits of fiber, antioxidants and phytonutrients, to name just a few.

This particular smoothie packs a wallop – forty-eight grams of protein (without the protein powder it would still have twenty-nine grams of protein) and it's very filling. This is well over fifty percent of what I require in a given day, so not bad for a breakfast or snack smoothie. If you want to know how many grams of protein you should eat in a given day, check out this blog on my website (*www.RootCauseMedicalClinics.com*) "How Much Protein do You Need?"

This smoothie can be changed up a bit (I provide options below) but if you want the high protein content – the soy milk, hemp seeds – my favorite is our Chocolate Vegan Protein Powder. Nut butter ingredients are the ones providing the high protein you need.

This smoothie isn't particularly sweet, so I give you the option of adding another banana and/or dates/date syrup to "up" the sweet quotient. This would be particularly good for kids or those gradually moving towards healthier eating.

This smoothie is about 400 to 450 calories – fine if you consider it a healthy, robust breakfast, but do realize it is a substantial part of your daily calorie consumption.

Let me know how you enjoy it!

Ingredients

- 1 cup unsweetened organic soy milk (8 grams of protein). (Option: You can use other plant-based milks if you prefer but the protein content will suffer.)

- 1 serving Balanced Plant-Based Protein Powder, your choice of vanilla or chocolate (20 grams of protein).

- 1 serving (2 to 3 tablespoons) organic hemp hearts (9-11 grams of protein).

- 1 tablespoon peanut butter (8 grams of protein). (Option: You can use other organic nut butters if you prefer, but your protein content will suffer.)

- 1 cup organic baby spinach (3 grams of protein).

- Optional for sweetness: 1 organic banana, 2 dates or 1 tablespoon date syrup

- Optional: A few ice cubes if you like your smoothies extra cold.

Method

- Place all ingredients except the protein powder in the blender and blend until completely smooth.

- Add the protein powder last and on low speed – just "stir" to combine. (This protein powder can get bitter if over-blended, hence best to add last.)

BANANA NUT PROTEIN SMOOTHIE

This is a protein-packed smoothie that will leave you satisfied for hours. Ingredients such as almonds, Brazil nuts and cinnamon are known to lower blood sugar, reduce cholesterol, protect your heart and are rich in antioxidants. They are also anti-inflammatory so other than throwing in a big handful of baby spinach or kale, this smoothie is hard to beat. Finally, it is thick and rich and so delicious you could call it a chocolate milkshake, and no one would know how healthy it was!

Ingredients

8 ounces organic almond milk

1 organic banana

1 serving Balanced Plant-Based Protein Powder, vanilla or chocolate

2 to 3 Brazil nuts

1 to 2 tablespoons of organic almond butter

1 teaspoon of cinnamon

1 tablespoon of cacao powder

Optional: Sweeten to taste using 1 to 2 teaspoons organic coconut sugar OR granulated monk fruit sweetener OR liquid stevia (SweetLeaf is best)

Method

• Blend together until smooth and enjoy!

AVOCADO BANANA SMOOTHIE

Personally, I LOVE avocados. A refrigerator with no avocados is something that MUST be addressed in my house. Similarly, I ADORE bananas. I'm rather particular (don't laugh too hard at this comment if you know me!) about said banana. Not too ripe, but just right, is the way I like it.

Therefore, with the two major ingredients being two of my favorite foods, you can only imagine how much I love this smoothie. I hope you do too.

Serves 2

Ingredients

1 cup canned organic unsweetened coconut milk, mixed well

½ cup organic unsweetened almond milk

1 organic avocado, ripe but not overripe

1 organic banana, ripe

Optional: Sweeten to taste using 1 to 2 teaspoons organic coconut sugar OR granulated monk fruit sweetener OR liquid stevia (SweetLeaf is best)

Strawberry variation:

Add 2 cups frozen organic strawberries (you could also try raspberries if you prefer them)

Additional ½ cup of organic unsweetened almond milk

Blueberry variation:

Add 2 cups of frozen organic blueberries

Additional ½ cup of organic unsweetened almond milk

Method

- Put all ingredients in a high-speed blender and blend until smooth and creamy. Enjoy!

VEGAN GOLDEN MILK SMOOTHIE

Golden milk is an ayurvedic medicine recipe (anti-inflammatory and immunity boosting). Traditionally it is prepared as a milk and served warm before bed to aid in sleep and the body's overnight restorative/repair process. Patients can omit the banana, almond butter, flax, and ice and they are left with a nice golden milk recipe that can be heated in a saucepan on the stovetop.

Serves 1 to 2

Ingredients

- 8 ounces unsweetened soy milk, almond milk (or other unsweetened non-dairy milk of choice)
- 1 medium-sized banana
- 2 tablespoons almond butter (or other nut butter of choice)
- 2 tablespoons golden flax meal
- 1 teaspoon ground ginger
- 1 teaspoon ground turmeric
- ½ teaspoon ground cinnamon
- Optional: ¼ teaspoon black pepper (helps the body readily absorb the turmeric)
- a pinch of pink Himalayan sea salt
- 1 to 2 teaspoons granulated monk fruit, date syrup or maple syrup (or ¼ teaspoon liquid stevia)
- 4 to 5 ice cubes

Method

- Combine all ingredients in blender and puree until smooth.

- Adjust seasonings and sweeteners to taste.

- For a thicker smoothie, feel free to add another ½ banana and/or additional almond butter (add by 1 tablespoon) and/or additional ice.

STRAWBERRIES AND CREAM SMOOTHIE

This is truly a luscious and pretty pink smoothie.

You can have fun making changes in the fruit or the type of milk you use, but it's pretty darn perfect just the way it is, in my opinion. Our health coach created this recipe and when we tasted it as a team, it got a unanimous "thumbs up!"

You can serve this to kids, omitting the fact that it's actually good for them! Believe me, they will never know how healthy it is based on the taste.

If you are trying to transition yourself or your family away from dairy products and you've been missing the creamy texture they provide, here's your solution.

You can substitute blueberries for red berries and enjoy a purple-blue vs. pink smoothie. You can also use a different plant-based milk such as almond or cashew if you prefer.

If the pure coconut cream gives you calorie concerns, stick with just the milk and realize it will be a bit less thick, but still delicious. You could also substitute ice to give it a thickness that way and reduce the fat and calorie count.

Play with the recipe and let us know any variations you enjoy!

Serves 4 to 6

Ingredients

2 medium sized ripe organic bananas, peeled

½ cup organic fresh raspberries, rinsed (frozen is an option)

10 ounces frozen organic strawberries

1 can (13.5 fl oz) of organic coconut milk

1 can (5.4 fl oz) of unsweetened organic coconut cream

1 tablespoon organic vanilla extract

SweetLeaf organic liquid stevia, to taste. (Five to ten drops can go a long way but keep tasting until it's where you like it.)

Method

- Place all ingredients in blender and blend until smooth (start on low and work up to higher speed.)

- Garnish with fresh fruit if desired e.g. fresh strawberries and/or raspberries. Serve immediately or refrigerate in an airtight container overnight for several hours.

- Best served within 24 hours to avoid discoloration from oxidation and enhance nutritional content.

STRAWBERRY PEACH KALE SMOOTHIE

Serves 2

Ingredients

2 cups unsweetened soy, almond, hemp, or coconut milk

1 cup frozen organic strawberries (no sugar added)

1 cup frozen organic peaches (no sugar added)

2 cups fresh organic kale

1 teaspoon vanilla extract

2 scoops vanilla protein powder (Balanced Plant-Based Protein Powder)

Method

- Put all in ingredients in a blender and mix well. Add ice to make smoothie more slushy, if desired.

- Tips: Healthy options include adding 1 tablespoon ground flax or chia seeds to add omega-3 fats and/or substituting organic baby spinach for the kale.

SNACKS

THE BEST ENERGY BITES!

I LOVE energy bites and I am a bit excited about this newest recipe! I find it very rewarding to make a super-fast, no-cook, healthy snack that keeps us all "munch happy" for the entire week. Although truth be told, I made these for the first time yesterday and barely two hours went by before I made batch two. Okay, we aren't pigs, but it was a Sunday, the basketball game was on, we'd taken a long hike in the morning, and you know what happened…

But seriously, it is so fun to make these and equally easy to change them up so they always taste different. If you are tired of peanut butter, try almond or cashew. If you are avoiding chocolate, use raisins or cranberries or even chopped walnuts.

Most recipes call for honey or maple syrup, but I tried date syrup, the healthiest sweetener available, and they were delicious. The date syrup is dark and imparts a slightly reddish-brown color to the balls.

I was also glad the ground flax worked so well because it is incredibly healthy for you. It's packed with fiber, anti-cancer, helps lower blood pressure and is just an all-around superfood.

For my next iteration I am going to make my own chocolate chunks with pure cacao and date syrup. I know, sounds extreme, but I want these one hundred percent sugar-free with still a cacao hit. I will keep you updated…

Let me know what combinations you come up with!

Serving size: 10 bites

Ingredients

1 cup gluten-free rolled oats

⅔ cup toasted organic coconut flakes

½ cup organic peanut butter or almond butter (If you use unsalted nut butter, consider adding a pinch of Himalayan sea salt.)

½ cup ground organic golden flax seeds

½ cup bittersweet chocolate chopped into chip-sized pieces (Option: use toasted organic walnuts or raisins or cranberries, if avoiding chocolate. Lily's chocolate chips are sweetened with stevia and are another alternative you can purchase. You can also make your own sugar-free chocolate. For the recipe, visit my website at *www. RootCauseMedicalClinics.com.*)

⅓ cup organic date syrup

1 teaspoon organic vanilla extract

Method

- Place all ingredients in a bowl and combine thoroughly.

- Refrigerate for about half an hour to make the dough hold together easier.

- Remove chilled dough from refrigerator and roll into 1″ bites.

- Place in airtight container and enjoy throughout the week.

CASHEW-DUSTED KALE CHIPS

Servings: 16 (1 serving ≈ ⅓ cup)

Ingredients

2 pounds organic dinosaur kale

¼ cup organic refined coconut oil

Optional: 1 tablespoon lemon juice

½ teaspoon sea salt

⅓ cup raw organic cashews, ground

1 tablespoon nutritional yeast

Method

- Preheat oven to 350° F (if baking in oven and not in a dehydrator).

- Strip the kale from the tough stems. Rinse thoroughly and dry. Tear or chop into smaller pieces and set aside.

- Make a dressing in a large bowl with the oil, lemon juice, and salt. Toss with kale to coat, then massage for about 1 minute to break down vegetable fibers.

- Sprinkle kale with ground nuts and nutritional yeast. Toss again.

- Place kale in a single layer on dehydrator sheets or baking pans. (Single layers provide the best results from dehydrating or baking. If kale is piled in more than one layer it will steam and not get crispy.)

- Dehydrate for two hours or according to dehydrator directions for greens.

- If baking in an oven, bake for 15 minutes until leaves are crispy and crunchy. Allow to cool completely before serving or storing in an airtight container.

- Tip: These kale chips turn out best in a dehydrator. Watch closely if baking in oven, as kale can burn easily.

EASY RAW ENERGY BITES

There are a lot of fruit and nut bars on the market. Some have good ingredients, but the liability of pre-packaging is that I find often the nuts have gone rancid. Training your taste buds to detect what a rancid oil tastes like is a good skill because rancid oils are dangerous.

Making this recipe at home allows for as much variety as you like. You can change up the type of dried fruit, nuts or nut butter you use. It's a quick, easy, fun recipe and the bites are packed with protein and healthy fat. A delicious, raw, vegan recipe for energy bites!

Ingredients

1 cup organic dates

1 cup organic raw pecans

½ cup organic shredded coconut

1 tablespoon organic peanut butter, no sugar added

1 tablespoon organic coconut oil

½ teaspoon organic vanilla

½ teaspoon sea salt

Method

- Soak dates in hot water for at least 10 minutes. Drain dates and add them to your food processor.

- Blend all ingredients in the food processor until it forms a dough. Roll into 12 small balls and refrigerate. That is it!

- Tip: You can always change it up by using different ingredients such as walnuts, raisins or prunes. You can even roll the energy bites in crushed sunflower seeds or raw cacao.

BAKED SWEET POTATO FRIES

Everyone loves fries. When the family first went gluten-free we were very upset to learn the number of restaurant French fries that contained gluten. The restaurants that did not offer coated fries definitely became our "best friends". But then we learned more about possible cross-contamination with gluten products used in the same fryers. And there was the realization that the oils used to fry the potatoes were re-used so often that they were very unhealthy and inflammatory.

Sweet potatoes have a higher nutritional value than white potatoes and, needless to say, baking rather than deep frying increases their health value as well.

When you need a great snack and are craving fries, enjoy these very healthy versions. These sweet potato fries are filling yet have none of the unhealthy ingredients of regular fries.

Ingredients

2 pounds of organic sweet potatoes, regular or purple variety

3 tablespoons of organic avocado oil or coconut oil

1 ½ teaspoons sea salt

1 ½ teaspoons organic coconut sugar or date sugar

¼ teaspoon cumin

¼ teaspoon chili powder

dash of cayenne

Method

- Preheat oven to 425°F.

- Peel the sweet potatoes and cut into wedges about the size and shape of steak fries.

- Mix the rest of the ingredients together in a bowl. Use a whisk or fork to fully combine.

- Pour the mixture over the cut fries and mix with your hands to get all the fries fully coated.

- Place the fries on a baking sheet, not touching each other and bake for fifteen minutes. Flip the fries over and bake for another fifteen minutes.

- Serve alone or with the condiment of your choice.

BEST HUMMUS RECIPE

Hummus seems like it would be so easy. You can "cheat" and get cooked garbanzo beans – that plus a food processor or blender should make the job quick and easy, right?

Well as much as I love hummus, I was having trouble finding a recipe that worked. There really are only a few ingredients in hummus, which confused me more as to why I could not make a version at home that my family and I loved.

Recently I have been cooking all my own beans from scratch to avoid any chemicals coming from boxes or cans. (I know, I am always taking it to the next level :-)

But my frustration grew as I made the effort to soak and cook garbanzos, only to have my family dislike the final product. I had to agree. I tried to "salvage" it with more lemon juice, etc., but no good.

Enter our patient Janette B. to save the day! Janette loves to cook, and we frequently exchange our new favorite recipes. She mentioned a new hummus recipe she had been enjoying, courtesy of her husband's cousin Patti. (And isn't that the way cooking should be – an exchange with friends and family of nourishing recipes that delight the palate AND keep us healthy?)

Kudos to Patti – this recipe is a keeper! She also shared a fun tip to make the hummus smoother, which I will admit I have not tried yet. It is listed in the method section below. Let me know what you think.

Serve this with some raw veggies such as cucumbers or carrots, or if you're in a healthy cracker mood, make up a batch of my

Crunchy Seed Crackers, which can be found on my website: *www.RootCauseMedicalClinics.com.*

Ingredients

1 cup cooked organic garbanzo beans (boxed or canned is fine)

¼ cup pure filtered water

Optional: 1 to 2 medium cloves organic garlic, depending on your garlic palate

1 tablespoon organic tahini

1 organic lemon, juiced (can use more to taste)

¼ teaspoon organic cumin

⅛ teaspoon cayenne pepper

Himalayan sea salt to taste

Method

- Open a can or box of garbanzo beans; rinse and drain thoroughly.

- Optional: Pour the beans into a saucepan with a cup or more of water plus 1 to 2 tablespoons of baking soda. Bring the beans to a boil and then let them stand for about twenty minutes. Pour the beans into a strainer and rinse them in cold water. This will separate the beans from the shells, making for a smoother hummus.

- Place the garlic into your food processor and pulse a few times to break it up.

- Add the rest of the ingredients plus about half the water and blend until very smooth. Add more water as needed to attain desired consistency. It will take about ¼ cup but start with half that and add more as needed.

- Season to taste.

- Put the hummus in a bowl and drizzle some olive oil and either paprika or cayenne pepper to give it a little color.

SPINACH AND ARTICHOKE DIP

You know how dips are – addicting, creamy deliciousness that it's all but impossible to stop eating. Historically, spinach artichoke dips are no different. The spinach and artichoke part makes it sound healthy, but then along comes the sour cream and cream cheese and all is lost.

Fear not, dip lovers. Our super smart registered dietitian has taken all the "bad" out of this traditional dip and left all the delicious creamy texture (while being plant-based). It's almost miraculous!

Enjoy this dip at your next dinner party, sports event or just as a nice appetizer for the family.

> **Note:** if onions and garlic "bother" you, substitute asofo-teida as recommended at the beginning of this chapter as a substitute.

Ingredients

- 1 can (14 oz) organic artichoke hearts, drained, rinsed & chopped
- 1 cup dairy-free parmesan "cheese"
- 1 container (5.3 oz) Kite Hill Greek-style yogurt
- 1 container (8 oz) of Kite Hill cream cheese
- Optional: 2 cloves of organic garlic, minced
- Optional: ½ organic yellow onion, diced
- 1 bag (5 oz) organic spinach
- 1 tablespoon organic avocado oil

Method

- Preheat oven to 350°F.

- In a skillet, add the avocado oil. Once warm, sauté the onion and garlic until tender.

- Add the spinach to the skillet, stirring until wilted.

- In a separate bowl, combine the Greek-style yogurt, cream cheese, artichoke hearts, and parmesan – save a small bit of parmesan to sprinkle over the top of the dish.

- Add the sautéed veggies to the mixture and stir well.

- Transfer the mixture to an 8×8" oven-safe pan, or the skillet used to sauté the veggies if it is oven-safe. Top with the remaining cheese and bake for twenty minutes.

- Serve with gluten-free Simple Mills crackers, carrots, or any raw vegetable of your choice.

HERBED WHITE BEAN DIP

Do not let the word "dip" fool you. While this could certainly be used as a dip alongside carrot, celery sticks, or the raw vegetable of your choice, it is also a great addition to a meal.

The beans make it high in protein as well as fiber, and the garlic gives it a flavor and health boost. Garlic is anti-inflammatory and anti-cancer and should be in your daily diet somewhere.

This dip is balanced with the right amount of protein, fiber and fat – you'll find it to be extremely filling. It is ridiculously easy to make and, like hummus, is something you can just have on hand for snacks as well as a bean side dish to any meal.

Do not be dismayed at the mild flavor when you first make it – the garlic takes about an hour or so to permeate fully. But then it is very flavorful and delicious.

Ingredients

  1 can organic cannellini beans, rinsed and drained

  ¼ cup organic avocado oil

  2 tablespoons water

  1 tablespoon organic lemon juice

  Optional: 2 cloves organic garlic

  ¼ cup organic fresh dill

  1 teaspoon Himalayan sea salt

  ½ teaspoon freshly ground pepper

Method

- Blend all the ingredients in a food processor until smooth. Adjust seasoning to taste. Enjoy with our crackers or raw vegetables!

HEALTHY SPRING ROLLS

(This recipe is my personal creation. There are many similar recipes online; I got inspiration from several but there is none exactly like this one... at least not that I know of!)

Happy Spring! Have you ever made spring rolls? I always thought they were something exclusive to eating out. They seemed as if they might be difficult to make and the sauce typically served with them tends to be pretty sweet, so I avoided it. But my smart daughter brought home spring roll "paper" and we began experimenting.

They are actually a lot of fun to make and you can use whatever healthy veggies you happen to have on hand. Think with colors of the rainbow so they are "pretty," not to mention healthy.

You can add sprouts, organic tofu, quinoa in addition to a variety of vegetables.

We had fun creating the sauce which, as made, is fairly spicy. You can avoid the Sriracha or simply cut down the amount to make a "tamer" version.

Please let me know how you enjoy these and any fun combinations you come up with.

Send me a picture and I will post it on my Instagram!

Servings: 4 to 8 rolls

Ingredients

rice paper

organic veggies, thinly sliced approximately 3″ in length. (Consider ¼ cup each of bell pepper, carrots, arugula, purple cabbage, green onions, avocado, or anything else you have on hand.)

squeeze of organic lemon

<u>Sauce</u>

½ cup organic peanut butter

¼ cup of garlic flavored coconut aminos

¼ cup of organic Tamari

1 tablespoon of Sriracha (use less if you want it less spicy)

Method

- Dip an individual rice paper in bowl of warm water for a couple seconds. Remove and place on a cutting board.

- Place prepared veggies into the middle, using about ⅓ to ½ cup total.

- Squeeze some fresh organic lemon juice over the veggies.

- Tuck the sides in towards the middle and roll.

- Whisk all the sauce ingredients in a bowl until smooth.

- Dip your spring roll in the sauce and enjoy!

NUT AND SEED BREAD

Baking bread is intimidating, at least in my opinion. Homemade bread typically involves yeast, allowing the dough to rise, etc., etc. This recipe is not difficult to make and if you have all the ingredients and a food processor, you can be enjoying this tasty treat in under two hours (cooking time is one hour).

I love bread but really do not tolerate grains very well. As soon as a grain is refined, I have issues, and I find many patients have similar problems. The refining of grains turns them into a simple carbohydrate that can spike insulin (blood sugar) and leave you with cravings for more simple carbs, including sugar.

Anything that offsets your blood sugar opens you up to craving the wrong foods, defeating all your hard work of trying to get healthy.

There are breads made from almond flour and eggs that are less refined, but it's still flour, and I don't like eggs as more than an occasional indulgence.

I created a similar bread a couple of years ago; you can see the recipe on my website: *www.RootCauseMedicalClinics.com*. It's similar, but my family and I like this one much better. Everyone's taste is different; see which you prefer and let me know.

Americans do not get enough fiber, but this bread will definitely tip the scales in the right direction. It is fiber-packed and VERY filling.

You can definitely "play" with the ingredients, changing up the nuts and seeds, substituting quinoa for oats, etc. If you make some changes, just try to keep the wet and dry measurements about the same so that the bread holds together well.

I liked the idea of dates vs. the maple syrup of the older recipe, since dates are a whole food and the dried cherries give a nice tang.

You will need a food processor for this recipe.

Ingredients

½ cup organic macadamia nuts (Option: try hazelnuts.)

½ cup organic almonds

1 cup organic sunflower seeds

½ cup organic pumpkin seeds

1 ½ cups organic and gluten-free rolled oats (Option: use quinoa flakes if you avoid oats.)

2 tablespoons organic chia seeds, ground

½ cup organic golden flax seeds, ground

4 tablespoons psyllium husk powder

1 teaspoon Himalayan sea salt

⅓ cup organic dates (approximately 4 dates), soaked

¼ cup organic dried cherries. (**Note:** These are a little tart; you can substitute raisins if you prefer.) Soak them with the dates.

3 tablespoons organic refined coconut oil, melted

2 cups water, warmed to about 100°F, divided into ½ and 1 ½ cups.

Method

- Preheat oven to 350°F (325°F if using convection)

- Take about four dates and the dried cherries and pour hot water over them, enough to cover completely. Let these sit about fifteen minutes while you're preparing the dry ingredients.

- Get a large mixing bowl and as you go through the below steps, add the ground nuts, seeds, etc. to the bowl.

- Place the almonds and macadamias in the processor and grind to a coarse flour. (Some chunks of nuts is totally fine – you do not want a finely ground flour.)

- Grind the seeds plus the oats, again to a coarse flour. (I leave it a little "chunky" with some bigger pieces of the seeds.)

- Grind the flax and chia together in a coffee grinder. You do want this fully ground up.

- Add all the above to a large mixing bowl.

- Last, add psyllium powder and salt and stir all the dry ingredients well to combine.

- Melt the coconut oil.

- Remove the stem and pit from the soaked dates and put them in your food processor along with ½ cup water. Blend until smooth.

- Set the soaked cherries aside.

- Heat the remaining 1 ½ cups water to about 100°F. Combine all the liquids and then add to the dry ingredients, stirring well to combine.

- Stir in the dried cherries.

- Line a glass bread pan with parchment paper.

- Press the dough into the dish. Ensure all air holes are removed from the dough and the top is flat.

- Cook at 350°F for 45 minutes.

- Remove from glass dish by simply pulling up on the parchment paper, then place directly on an oven rack or pizza pan dish for the remaining 15 minutes. (It's okay to leave the parchment paper attached.)

- Remove from oven and allow to completely cool on a cooling rack.

- Fresh from the oven the bread is delicious; after cooling toasting is best in my opinion.

- Enjoy!

- Loaf will keep about four days in the refrigerator. If you don't think you'll eat it that fast, slice and place in the freezer in individual plastic bags.

PUMPKIN BREAD

Fall is coming and everything "pumpkin" is in the air. There is something about the aroma of pumpkin, cinnamon, nutmeg, and cloves that harkens back to Thanksgiving morning and just makes you feel good. This pumpkin bread is delicious – it not only tastes delicious and smells delicious, it is *almost* perfect.

Almost? Well if you know me, I hold my recipes to very high standards. They must be fast, delicious AND uber-healthy. This bread does contain refined flours – potato, rice, etc., not my favorite. With that said, it still has a lot going for it – gluten-free, dairy-free, sugar-free, and vegan is pretty darn good. It could also be made nut-free very easily.

Serve it to anyone. It's moist, lightly sweet and your guests will never know it's healthy! Let me know how you enjoy it.

Prep time: 10 mins

Cook/Chill Time: 55 mins

Serving size: 1 loaf

Ingredients

1 can/box (15 oz) organic pumpkin puree (not pumpkin pie filling, just pure pumpkin)

⅓ cup organic avocado oil or refined organic coconut oil

⅔ cup organic maple syrup

2 teaspoons organic vanilla extract

1 tablespoon organic cinnamon

¼ teaspoon cloves

⅛ teaspoon nutmeg

dash of Himalayan sea salt

2 cups Bob's Red Mill all-purpose gluten-free flour mix, or mix of your choice

2 tablespoons coconut flour

1 ½ teaspoons gluten-free baking powder

1 teaspoon baking soda

1 teaspoon xanthan gum

1 cup total of add-ins – try organic raisins, chopped cashews, pumpkin seeds, and chopped dark chocolate bar. You can also make your own sugar-free chocolate by visiting my website at www.RootCauseMedicalClinics.com. Lily's chocolate chips are sweetened with stevia and can be purchased.

Optional: 1 tablespoon extra pumpkin seeds for garnish

Method

- Preheat oven to 350°F. Line a bread loaf pan with some oil and set aside.

- Place pumpkin puree, oil, maple syrup, vanilla extract, spices, and salt into a large mixing bowl and blend together using an immersion blender, regular blender, or mixer. Transfer into a medium mixing bowl.

- Add in all remaining ingredients, except for the add-ins and extra pumpkin seeds. Mix thoroughly with a wooden spoon to combine.

- Fold in the one cup of add-ins.

- Transfer the mixture into the bread loaf pan and smooth out. Very gently tap the pan on the counter a few times to eliminate any air bubbles. (If you tap too hard all the add-ins will sink to the bottom.) Sprinkle with pumpkin seeds on top.

- Bake in a preheated oven for about 55 to 60 minutes. (My convection oven had it cooked in 45 minutes, so start checking a little early for doneness.)

- Test with a wooden toothpick down the center to make sure it comes out dry. Once baked, let it cool for at least ten minutes prior to serving.

SOUPS

BUTTERNUT SQUASH SOUP

Learn how to make an easy dairy-free gluten-free organic roasted butternut squash apple soup with curry. Delicious, healthy, hearty, and filled with antioxidants and vitamins. I hope you enjoy this recipe!

Ingredients

1 organic butternut squash, cut into equal sized pieces

Optional: 2 medium organic yellow onions, quartered

2 organic Fuji apples, quartered

3 tablespoons of avocado or almond oil

2 to 4 cups of organic vegetable stock

½ to one teaspoon organic curry powder to taste (I used ⅜ for kids)

Condiments for serving:

¼ cup organic cashews, toasted and chopped

¼ cup organic shredded coconut, lightly toasted

Method

- Preheat oven to 425°F.

- Cut squash, onions, and apple in equal sizes and put into roasting pan.

- Pour oil over everything and mix it together, making sure everything is evenly covered in oil. Add salt and pepper to taste.

- Place in convection oven for 25 minutes total. Halfway through (approx. 12 minutes) turn over ingredients to make sure nothing is burning.

- Chop up cashews and add to pan over low heat with shredded coconut until aromatic – watch carefully to prevent burning.

- Meanwhile, heat the vegetable stock to a simmer.

- When the vegetables are done, put them through a food processor fitted with a steel blade.

- Add some of the vegetable stock and coarsely puree. When all the vegetables are processed, place them in a large pot and add enough vegetable stock to make a thick soup.

- Add the curry powder and add salt and pepper to taste.

- Reheat and serve hot with condiments either on the side or on top of each serving.

- You can always add some rice or enjoy this dairy-free gluten-free recipe by itself!

VEGETABLE BEAN SOUP

If it is a little cold outside, nothing is more warming and satisfying than soup. If you do not regularly cook at home, the concept of making soup from scratch can seem a little intimidating. Truly, nothing could be easier.

While this recipe calls for an Instant Pot (pressure cooker) or Crock Pot (slow cooker), if you do not have one it is totally fine. Start with sautéing the onions and garlic until softened and then follow the rest of the instructions below. If you are cooking on the stovetop, consider cutting the sweet potato into small bite-size pieces to decrease cooking time.

Further, if you do not have the time to soak dried beans overnight, you can simply use canned; just drain the liquid from the can before adding to the soup.

With small pieces of potato, the finished product should not take longer than what the Instant Pot takes: about 35 minutes.

Enjoy and let us know any variations you come up with.

(Adapted from One Lovely Life.)

Ingredients

- 1 lb. dry organic great northern beans (Option: canned organic beans)
- 2 teaspoons organic avocado oil
- Optional: 1 yellow organic onion, diced
- Optional: 2 cloves organic garlic, minced
- 3 organic carrots, diced

3 stalks organic celery, diced

1 large organic sweet potato, diced

1 can (15 oz) organic diced tomatoes

1 teaspoon organic oregano

½ teaspoon organic sage

½ teaspoon sea salt

4 cups organic veggie broth

Optional: 1 bag Quorn Chik'n Tenders to boost protein. (This is a mushroom-based vegetarian product with a small amount of egg white.)

Method

- Soak the beans in water overnight: place them in a large bowl with enough filtered water to cover them by 2 to 3 inches. The next day drain the beans and rinse well with filtered water.

- Turn the Instant Pot on the sauté setting and sauté the onion and garlic with the avocado oil until tender.

- Place the carrots, celery, onion, sweet potato, and tomatoes in the Instant Pot, then add the soaked and drained beans.

- Cover with broth and stir in spices.

- Turn Instant Pot to the pressure cook setting and cook for 35 minutes.

- If you do not have a pressure cooker, sauté the onion and garlic on the stove-top, then transfer to a Crock Pot with the remaining ingredients. Cook on low for 7 to 8 hours, or high for 3 to 4 hours.

SWEET GREEN PEA AND ASPARAGUS SOUP

Spring is a great time to enjoy all the green, healthy vegetables so prevalent during the season. This soup is delicious, nutritious, and beautiful (if you like the color green!).

Soups are easy to make and I love that you can easily double or triple the recipe and freeze some for a quick future meal. This soup is delicious warm but can be served cold or at room temperature if it is warm outside.

Asparagus is a good source of fiber and is a natural diuretic. It is full of vitamin K1, vitamin E, C and A plus healthy antioxidants and is rich in anti-inflammatory properties. Peas too are rich in vitamins, minerals and fiber, making this soup a powerhouse of nutrition.

You can serve this soup with a healthy salad and a side of beans or legumes to get a nice protein content. Also consider adding some fat with avocado, making it a "green sweep"!

Let me know how you enjoy this soup and any variations you enjoy.

This soup is modified elimination diet-friendly, so if you are a new patient this one is good to try.

Enjoy!

Serves 4 to 6.

Ingredients

   2 tablespoons organic avocado oil

   Optional: 1 medium organic yellow onion, chopped

   16 ounces organic asparagus (~3 cups trimmed into 1" pieces)

Optional: 2 to 3 cloves of garlic, minced

1 ½ teaspoons pink Himalayan sea salt, plus more to taste

1 teaspoon fresh cracked black pepper, plus more to taste

5 cups organic vegetable stock

6 ounces organic frozen sweet green peas, defrosted (~1 ½ to 2 cups)

¼ cup fresh tarragon, chopped

Optional: 2 tablespoons organic lemon juice

Method

- In a medium-sized pot, heat the avocado oil over medium heat. Add chopped yellow onion and cook for 3 to 4 minutes until translucent.

- Add trimmed asparagus, minced garlic, sea salt, and black pepper. Cook for another 3 to 4 minutes.

- Add vegetable stock and bring to gentle boil. Once boiling, reduce heat to a simmer and cook uncovered for 15 minutes.

- Add sweet green peas and tarragon, simmer for another 2 to 3 minutes.

- Remove from heat and cool for 5 minutes.

- Use an immersion blender, or transfer contents of pot to a blender with a secure lid. Blend until soup is completely pureed and smooth. (Pureeing in batches may be helpful if you are using a smaller sized blender)

- Return to pot and add lemon juice if using. Stir to combine and adjust sea salt and black pepper to taste.

- Serve warm.

- Garnish options: Fresh tarragon, sautéed asparagus spears and vegan parmesan (try Parma Alternative Vegan Parmesan Cheese, which is made with nutritional yeasts, nuts, and seeds AND is compliant with the elimination diet).

IMMUNITY-BOOSTING BEAN SOUP

This recipe was inspired by the Minimalist Vegan. The recipe comes from a soup her mother often made when she was not feeling well. As I am apt to do with most recipes, I have made a few modifications to it. I made it last night and it was a hit for my family.

This soup has some incredibly healthy ingredients including ginger, garlic, turmeric and kale – all known to be powerful immune boosters.

You can use pretty much any legume you like or happen to have on hand. You can try lentils, or even a combination of beans like cannellini and garbanzos.

That is one nice thing about making soup: you can use up things you have on hand.

This is a great soup to eat when you feel run down, need to warm up or are sick. Adding some more ginger, turmeric and garlic will help to pick your immune system up even more when you are unwell.

Ingredients

> ¼ cup extra-virgin olive oil
>
> Optional: 1 red (or yellow) organic onion, diced
>
> Optional: 4 organic garlic cloves, minced or finely chopped
>
> 2 to 3 medium organic carrots, diced
>
> 1 ½ to 2 tablespoons organic ginger, finely grated
>
> 4 cups cooked beans or lentils (If using from a can, rinse the beans thoroughly. I used mostly cannellini and 1 can garbanzo.)

½ to 1 teaspoon organic turmeric powder

6 cups vegetable broth

1 small bunch organic kale, roughly chopped (about 2 to 3 cups)

salt and pepper to taste

Method

- In a large saucepan, heat the oil and onion on medium until onion has become translucent.

- Add in the garlic and cook for another 1 to 2 minutes.

- Next add the carrots, ginger, beans and turmeric, cooking for an additional 5 to 7 minutes.

- Once the ingredients are well combined, pour in the vegetable broth.

- Bring to a boil and simmer for 10 minutes.

- Add in the kale and season to taste.

- Once the kale softens a little, the soup is ready.

VEGETABLE SOUP

My mother, a great cook, used to spend an entire day making split pea soup. No wonder I never liked to cook when young; I thought everything took an entire day to make!

Making soup from scratch can sound daunting but this recipe proves it does not have to be. My husband calls this my "refrigerator soup" because it changes depending on what I have on hand. That is true but it also means your family won't get bored!

The key to a healthy meal is ensuring you have a nice balance of nutrients and opting for those particular vegetables that are superfoods in their own right. These particular "gems" of the plant kingdom boast anti-inflammatory properties, they are anti-cancer and filled to the brim with healthy nutrients. What more can you ask from dinner?

Please let me know how you enjoy this and any varieties you come up with that you enjoy.

Ingredients

1 tablespoon organic avocado oil

Optional: 1 medium organic onion, finely chopped

Optional: 1 clove of organic garlic, finely chopped

½ cup red lentils, washed and picked over to remove any rocks

2 organic carrots, sliced

2 organic stalks of celery, sliced

Optional: 2 cans (10 oz) chopped organic tomatoes

1 quart organic vegetable broth

2 cups chopped organic kale, ribs removed

½ teaspoon organic oregano

salt and pepper to taste

Optional: 1 bag of Quorn Chik'n Tenders or 1 can organic cannellini beans.

Method

- To a large saucepan over medium heat, add oil.

- Once the oil is warm, sauté the onions and garlic until transparent, about 3 to 4 minutes.

- Add the lentils to the saucepan and stir to coat with the oil.

- Next add the carrots and celery and sauté for an additional 3 to 4 minutes. If anything is starting to stick, splash with some vegetable broth.

- Add the chopped tomatoes and vegetable broth, stirring to combine all the ingredients.

- Add the oregano, salt and pepper, stir once more and allow to simmer (covered) for about 10 minutes more.

- If you are going to add the Quorn or beans, do so now, then continue to cook about 4 minutes more. If not, add the kale now, stir and taste for seasoning.

- Once the kale has wilted into the soup you are done! I like my vegetables with a bit of "tooth" but if you want to cook them longer you can.

LENTIL SOUP

There is nothing like soup when it is cold outside. I particularly love soups that are a complete meal in one satisfying bowl.

If you are trying to eat a higher plant-based diet, which you should, this lentil soup delivers in a big way. The lentils provide protein, the kale is an amazing green, and it has healthy fat.

It is not only delicious and easy to prepare, but it is satisfying to even the largest appetites. When eating healthy, this is what you want – something that's so good and filling that you will not want anything "bad" to eat.

The flavors make it seem like it took hours to prepare when it is fully ready to eat in about 45 minutes. Enjoy this fast and easy vegan lentil soup.

(Soup has been adapted from a lentil soup by Cookie and Kate.)

Servings: 5 bowls of soup

Ingredients

¼ cup organic tea seed oil, avocado or coconut oil

Optional: 1 medium organic yellow chopped

2 organic carrots, peeled and chopped

Optional: 4 organic garlic cloves, pressed or minced

½ teaspoon organic dried thyme

Optional: 1 can (28 oz) organic diced tomatoes, or equivalent amount of fresh diced tomatoes

1 cup brown or green lentils, picked over and rinsed

5 cups organic vegetable broth

1 teaspoon salt, more to taste

Optional: A pinch red pepper flakes

freshly ground black pepper, to taste

2 cups chopped organic kale, ribs removed

Optional: Juice of ½ to 1 medium organic lemon, to taste

Method

- Warm the oil in a large Dutch oven or deep pot over medium heat. Once the oil is warm, add the chopped onion and carrot and cook, stirring often, until the onion has turned translucent, about 4 to 5 minutes.

- Add the garlic and thyme. Stir well for only a minute until fragrant.

- Pour in the diced tomatoes and cook for a few more minutes, stirring often so that all the flavors blend.

- Pour in the lentils and broth. Add 1 teaspoon salt and a pinch of red pepper flakes and season with freshly ground black pepper.

- Raise heat and bring the mixture to a gentle boil, then partially cover the pot and reduce heat to maintain a simmer.

- Cook for about 30 minutes total, or until the lentils are just tender. (Don't overcook the lentils or they'll fall apart.)

- Stir occasionally and after about 25 minutes of cooking, add the chopped kale.

- If you're adding lemon juice, do so once the soup is fully cooked.

- Taste and season with more salt, pepper and/or lemon juice.

CAULIFLOWER SOUP

When you think of "creamy" and "rich" soups, butter, cream and flour typically come to mind. But this wonderful recipe truly is creamy and rich along with being vegan, gluten-free and easy! Hopefully, it will become your choice for a warm, filling, and healthy soup.

It doesn't take much time to prepare (always a plus), and the ingredients can readily be found in your local markets.

Often recipes for a thick and creamy soup require blending, but in this recipe the "thickness" comes from vegan cream or plant-based milk. The addition of lemon juice gives it a nice tang.

Each and every ingredient is particularly healthy and immune boosting plus anti-inflammatory.

Please let us know how you enjoy it!

Ingredients

  1 large organic cauliflower

  Optional: 1 large organic onion (any color will do)

  Optional: 3 cloves organic garlic

  1 teaspoon organic thyme, fresh or dried

  ¼ cup vegan butter (This adds a richness to the soup. Our current favorite is from Miyokos.) (Optional: substitute with avocado or olive oil)

  5 cups water or organic veggie broth

1 cup vegan cream. Options: Coconut cream (discard the water of a small can of full fat coconut milk), or a store-bought vegan cream, or your favorite plant-based milk. Oat milk would do nicely as well.)

1 small organic lemon, juiced

salt and pepper to taste

Method

- Dice the onion and mince the garlic cloves.

- Cut the cauliflower into bite-size florets. Discard the thick stem.

- Sauté the onion in vegan butter or avocado oil in a heavy-bottom pan over medium heat until the onions begin to caramelize – about 5 to 6 minutes.

- Add the garlic and cook 1 minute more.

- Add remaining ingredients: cauliflower, thyme, salt, pepper and water.

- Bring the soup to a boil, cover and reduce heat, simmer for twenty minutes.

- Remove from the heat and stir in the vegan cream or plant milk plus the lemon juice.

- Let the soup rest for ten minutes to cool.

- Option: You can enjoy the soup now, or if you prefer it creamier, you can use an immersion blender or cup blender, pureeing the soup until desired consistency.

- Some people prefer a half-blended version where there are still some chunks of cauliflower remaining.

- Reheat on the stove if needed to warm back up before serving.

- And now you're ready to enjoy!

- (This version of vegan cauliflower soup is courtesy of Simple Veganista.)

VEGAN CREAM OF BROCCOLI SOUP

It takes only five ingredients and thirty minutes to make this "cream" of broccoli soup. It is delicious and will fill you up, plus it's packed with antioxidants and good-for-you greens!

Ingredients

2 tablespoons organic oil (avocado, tea seed or coconut)

Optional: 1 large organic onion sliced

1 head of organic broccoli or cauliflower, cut into florets; stalk peeled if tough and cut into pieces

Optional: 2 cloves of garlic, chopped

salt and pepper to taste

Optional: ½ cup of white wine

3 cups organic vegetable broth

1 cup cashew cream (recipe below) or coconut milk

Method

- Put the oil in a large, deep saucepan on medium heat. Once the oil is heated, add the onion, broccoli, garlic, salt, and pepper. Cook until the onion is transparent, about 10 minutes.

- Add the wine if you're using it and cook another minute or two.

- Add the vegetable broth and cook until the broccoli is tender, about 10 minutes.

- Let the soup cool enough that it is safe to put it into a blender, then blend until it reaches the consistency you like.

- Add the cashew cream* or coconut milk, reheat as needed, season to taste and serve.

- *Cashew Cream Recipe

- Take ¾ cup of organic raw cashews and ½ to ¾ cup of purified water and blend on high speed until you have a smooth consistency. You can make the cream thicker or thinner by using more of less water.

- Soaking cashews for about thirty minutes beforehand will speed up the process. You will need a high-speed blender to make the milk. If you don't have one, then soak the cashews for several hours or overnight by just covering them with water. This will soften them and make them much easier to blend.

- To watch my video demonstration for this recipe, visit my website at: *www.RootCauseMedicalClinics.com.*

ENTREES

GREEK LENTIL STEW

Servings: 4

Ingredients

1 tablespoon extra-virgin organic olive oil

Optional: 1 small organic red onion, chopped

1 medium organic yellow sweet pepper, chopped

Optional: 2 cloves organic garlic, finely chopped

1 cup organic lentils (red lentils cook the fastest)

2 teaspoons dried oregano

1 teaspoons ground cinnamon

2½ cups low-sodium organic vegetable broth, divided

1 medium organic zucchini squash, chopped

1 medium organic yellow squash, chopped

1 tablespoon organic tomato paste

½ cup unsweetened pomegranate juice

½ teaspoon sea salt

¼ teaspoon black pepper

Method

- In a small Dutch oven, heat oil over medium-high heat. Add onion and bell pepper, and sauté for one minute. Cover pot tightly and cook over medium heat for four minutes.

- Add garlic and cook for one minute longer.

- Stir in lentils, oregano, and cinnamon, and cook until seasoning is fragrant, about 30 seconds.

- Add 2 cups of broth. Bring to a boil, reduce heat and cover. Simmer lentils for 25 minutes.

- Add zucchini and yellow squash, tomato paste, pomegranate juice, remaining broth, sea salt and

- pepper. Simmer for 15 minutes, or until lentils are done to your taste.

- Let stew sit, uncovered, for 15 minutes. Serve warm or at room temperature, divided among

- soup bowls.

KALE SALAD

Servings: 6 (1 serving ≈ 1 cup)

Ingredients

1 bunch organic kale

½ teaspoon sea salt

Optional: ¼ cup diced red onion

⅓ cup currants, raisins, or dried cranberries or cherries (no sugar added)

⅓ cup diced apple (about ½ an apple)

⅓ cup sunflower seeds, toasted

¼ cup olive oil

2 teaspoons red wine vinegar or unfiltered apple cider vinegar

Method

- De-stem kale by pulling leaves away from stems. Wash leaves, then spin or pat dry. Stack the leaves, roll them up and cut into thin ribbons. Put kale in a large mixing bowl.

- Add salt and massage it into the kale with your hands for two minutes (skipping this step will leave you with tough, stringy kale.)

- Stir onions with dried fruit, apple, and sunflower seeds into the kale.

- Dress with oil and vinegar.

- Taste for sea salt and vinegar, adding more if necessary. Also taste a few bites to see if balance of sweet/sour/ crunchy/chewy are all well mixed. Add extra of whatever you want.

ROASTED ROOT VEGETABLE SALAD

Makes 4 servings

Ingredients

- 1 medium organic sweet potato (about 4 ounces), cut into ¾" cubes
- 1 medium organic yellow potato, cut into ¾" cubes (Option: substitute parsnip.)
- 1 medium organic carrot, peeled, cut into ¾" slices
- Optional: 1 small organic red onion, cut into ½" wedges
- 2 medium organic celery stalks, cut into ¾" slices
- 1 medium organic beet, cut into ¾" cubes
- 1 ½ tablespoons extra-virgin olive oil, divided
- ¼ teaspoon sea salt
- ¼ teaspoon freshly ground black pepper
- 1 teaspoon balsamic vinegar
- Optional: 2 teaspoons fresh lemon juice
- ½ teaspoon Dijon mustard
- 1 tablespoon fresh parsley, chopped
- 1 teaspoon fresh cilantro, chopped
- 2 tablespoons organic walnuts, finely chopped

Method

- Preheat oven to 425° F.

- In a large bowl, toss together the potatoes (sweet and yellow), carrot, red onion, celery, beet, and ½ tablespoon of the oil, coating well. Season with sea salt and pepper.

- Arrange vegetables on a cookie sheet and spread mixture evenly in a single layer.

- Roast, stirring several times, until tender and beginning to brown, about 50 minutes.

- In a small bowl, whisk together vinegar, lemon juice, and Dijon mustard with remaining tablespoon of oil, and stir in parsley and cilantro. Drizzle dressing over vegetables, add walnuts, and gently toss.

Serve warm or at room temperature.

CASHEW "CHEESE" SAUCE

Many recipes call for a cheese sauce. It is also a fun addition to many vegetable dishes. But when you are avoiding dairy products you start to feel like such a creamy indulgence is completely off limits.

This easy, healthy recipe is creamy and delicious, and you won't miss the dairy.

Ingredients

1 ¼ cups of organic raw cashews

½ cup of nutritional yeast

2 tablespoons of organic lemon juice

½ organic vegetable bouillon cube, dissolved in warm water

3 cups of organic almond milk

½ cup of organic avocado oil or tea seed oil

½ cup of agar-agar flakes

Seasonings:

Optional: 2 teaspoons organic onion powder

2 teaspoons sea salt

Optional: 1 teaspoon garlic powder

⅛ teaspoon ground black pepper

Method

- Combine the almond milk, oil and agar-agar flakes in a saucepan over medium heat and heat until agar-agar has fully dissolved and the mixture has thickened. Once the milk and agar mixture has thickened, take it off the heat.

- Pulse the cashews in the food processor until finely ground, but do not let it turn into cashew butter. Add all seasonings plus nutritional yeast to the food processor. Pulse a couple of times to combine.

- Start the food processor and while its running, slowly add the agar-agar. Continue running the processor until the mixture is smooth and creamy.

- Add ¼ cup of hot water to the bouillon cube to make it into a broth. Add the lemon juice and bouillon broth to the food processor. Pulse a couple of times to gently combine.

- Your vegan cashew "cheese" is ready to eat! You can enjoy it warm over gluten-free pasta for "mac and cheese" or add it to a Mexican inspired dish with salsa.

- Whatever "cheese" you don't use immediately, put in the refrigerator in a glass dish to solidify. Once it has cooled you can slice it or shred it for anything you would use regular cheese for.

- Keeps for a week in the refrigerator.

SPRING QUINOA SALAD AND BASIL VINAIGRETTE

Do you like quinoa? If you haven't tried it I urge you to do so. This particular recipe is so full of flavor you won't even notice the quinoa if it's a new addition to your diet.

Quinoa is often prepared and spoken about as if it is a grain, when in fact it is a seed.

It is a member of the spinach, chard and beet family – perhaps that's why it's so good for you. It has a good protein profile and is loaded with nutrients and vitamins. Quinoa is a complete protein, containing all the essential (nine) amino acids. Plus it provides a majority of the essential nutrients required for life. It's estimated that no food is better than quinoa in this regard.

It is naturally gluten-free and there are over one hundred different varieties.

This particular recipe is very filling and delicious. It's very easy to make and you can do a variety of things with it.

I enjoyed having it with arugula, although any lettuce would do. Please let me know how you enjoy this recipe and any fun variations you come up with.

Thanks goes out to our Health Coach who created this recipe.

Serves 4 to 8

Ingredients

½ cup uncooked organic quinoa, rinsed in cool water

16 ounces frozen organic petite green peas

Optional: ½ chopped large organic shallot

½ cup chopped fresh organic Italian parsley

½ cup crumbled Kite Hill vegan ricotta cheese

½ cup chopped organic walnuts

<u>Basil vinaigrette</u>

1 cup packed organic basil leaves, chopped

½ cup organic avocado oil OR extra-virgin olive oil

½ small to medium organic shallot

Optional: 1 medium organic garlic clove

1 scant tablespoon pure organic maple syrup

3 tablespoons organic white wine vinegar

Optional: 1 pinch red pepper flakes

Himalayan sea salt and fresh cracked black pepper, to taste

Method

- In a medium saucepan, prepare quinoa according to package instructions, fluff, and set aside. Optional: Use organic vegetable broth in place of water for additional flavor. This is what I do when I cook quinoa.

- While waiting for the quinoa to cook, heat a large pot of boiling water.

- In a medium bowl, create an ice water bath.

- Blanch the frozen green peas by putting them into the boiling water for 1 to 2 minutes, or until the peas turn bright green and are warmed through.

- Drain in a colander and quickly drop the peas into the ice water bath to stop the cooking process. Drain the ice water and set the peas aside.

- In a medium-large serving bowl, combine the fluffed quinoa, peas, shallot, parsley, ricotta cheese, and walnuts.

Basil Vinaigrette

- In a blender, combine basil, avocado oil, shallot, garlic, maple syrup, white wine vinegar, red pepper flakes (if using), and a pinch of sea salt and black pepper.

- Blend until the dressing is smooth.

- Adjust salt and pepper to taste.

Assembly

- Toss ¾ of the dressing in with the quinoa salad and adjust with additional dressing, salt, and pepper to taste.

HIGH PROTEIN VEGGIE PASTA

When you think of veggies and pasta, it sounds like a heavy carbohydrate meal. Granted, the veggies are good complex carbs, but what about pasta?

Traditionally, wheat or even rice pasta is a high refined carbohydrate and will often leave you feeling hungry quickly and craving sugar. That is definitely not what we're going for with our healthy eating plans.

What if there was a pasta that was delicious and had none of the simple carbohydrate liabilities? What if a serving of pasta had more protein than a burger or chicken breast? Sounds incredible but the market for healthy, high protein pasta has spoken and manufacturers have provided great options.

In this recipe we feature the lentil-based Tolerant pasta, but you can also try garbanzo bean-based Banza pasta. Both provide over twenty grams of healthy plant-based protein per serving. They are easy to cook and delicious.

If you've missed pasta because you are gluten-free or just intolerant to refined carbohydrates, your pasta prayers have been answered!

This recipe is a great easy lunch or dinner that's gluten-free and plant-based while being full of protein and healthy vegetables.

Ingredients

1 box Banza high-protein pasta

2 cups of organic broccoli, chopped into small florets

1 cup organic cherry tomatoes, quartered

1 organic bell pepper, chopped

Optional: ¼ cup organic finely diced red onion

4 tablespoons extra-virgin olive oil

2 tablespoons red wine vinegar

Optional: 1 clove organic garlic, minced

¼ teaspoon salt

1 teaspoon Italian seasoning

Method

- Prep pasta according to package instructions and let it cool.
- Chop veggies and combine with pasta.
- Combine oil, vinegar, garlic & spices. Whisk to combine.
- Pour over pasta salad and serve

BUTTERNUT SQUASH RISOTTO

Risotto is a traditional rich, delicious, creamy side dish that's typically made with plenty of butter, flour and cheese. Despite that traditional preparation, you can enjoy this recipe without any worry if you are avoiding dairy and/or gluten.

What I love about this recipe is that it "screams" traditional risotto while avoiding the negative ingredients completely.

You can confidently serve this to guests and they'll be none the wiser about its healthy ingredients. They will probably notice they feel better after eating it, however!

The color and texture of this dish makes it a perfect addition to your Thanksgiving and holiday table. Your loved ones and guests can enjoy this vitamin-packed side dish, worry free.

Ingredients

2 tablespoons vegan butter or extra-virgin olive oil

Optional: 4 cloves organic garlic, minced

Optional: 2 stalks organic green onions

2 cups organic Arborio rice

½ cup dry white wine or veggie broth

6 cups organic veggie broth of your choice

1 medium organic butternut squash (about 3 to 4 cups cubed)

1 tablespoon olive oil

1 tablespoon poultry seasoning or sage

Optional, for color: ⅛ teaspoon turmeric

2 tablespoon extra-virgin olive oil

salt and pepper to taste

Method

- Wash the squash and place it in the oven at 300°F for about 30 minutes, until it becomes slightly soft. Remove from the oven and let it cool until you can hold it.

- Peel and cube the squash. Place cubes on a cookie sheet and sprinkle with olive oil, salt, and pepper.

- Bake the cubes at 375° F for 30 minutes, flipping with a spatula every 10 minutes until slightly crisp on the outside.

- While the squash is baking, add 6 cups of veggie broth to a medium saucepan, and add a tablespoon of poultry seasoning or sage to the broth. Heat and stir until the broth is warm.

- Also, while the cubed squash is baking, melt vegan margarine on low in a large pot.

- Add minced garlic and thinly sliced green onions. Warm for about 3 minutes in the margarine.

- Pour in 2 cups Arborio rice (dry unwashed) and coat the rice with butter and garlic. It will turn slightly translucent.

- Add the wine (or ½ cup of broth) and stir until it absorbs.

- Add remaining 6 cups of broth mixture about ½ a cup at a time, never adding more until the liquid has been absorbed.

- Stir slowly and constantly, adding more broth each time the liquid is absorbed, being careful not to let the rice burn at the bottom of the pot. (Risotto requires your full attention!)

- When all the broth has been used up, turn off the heat and add the roasted squash to the rice and stir carefully until mixed.

- Serve immediately. Sprinkle with vegan Parmesan if desired.

- (Shout out to the vegan culinary blog "The Hidden Veggies" for sharing this recipe. Minor changes were made to the original recipe.)

ORGANIC KALE AND AVOCADO SALAD

This is a super healthy, delicious and easy kale salad that is loaded with great nutrition including protein!

Ingredients

1 small bunch organic dinosaur kale (or your kale of choice), washed, with inner rib removed

1 organic avocado, or more depending on your taste

Optional: 1 organic shallot finely chopped. May use raw or after lightly sautéing.

1 organic lemon, juiced

2 tablespoons nutritional yeast

1 to 2 teaspoons organic extra-virgin cold pressed olive oil

Optional: organic chickpeas for that added protein

Method

- Massage the kale beginning with 1 teaspoon of olive oil and a dash or two of salt. The kale will soften and turn a more vibrant green once it is fully massaged. It will be smiling too! LOL

- Cut the kale into bite-sized pieces and place in a medium salad bowl.

- Slice the avocado and mash it with a fork in a small bowl until it becomes a paste. Add the lemon juice to the avocado paste and mix.

- Now add the shallot, either raw or lightly sautéed.

- Add in the kale and mix well.

- Sprinkle the nutritional yeast on top, add the chickpeas and combine.

- At this point taste the salad and decide if you want to add more lemon juice or nutritional yeast, salt or pepper, depending on your taste.

- You can serve this salad with a warm entree, veggie burger or all by itself.

CHICKPEA LETTUCE WRAPS

If you are searching for healthy lunches and snacks for your family, give this a try! This recipe is full of plant-based protein and fiber. The lettuce-wrapped option leaves you feeling energized and full of nutrients.

Ingredients

2 cans organic chickpeas

5 stalks organic celery, finely diced (1 cup)

Optional: ⅓ cup scallions, sliced

3 large organic carrots, finely diced (1 cup)

1 container (5.3 oz) Kite Hill Greek-style almond milk yogurt (about 1 cup)

juice from half of a lemon

½ cup cashews, broken into pieces

¼ teaspoon paprika

¼ teaspoon salt

1 tablespoon curry powder

Optional: lettuce cups for serving

Method

- Drain & rinse chickpeas.
- Chop veggies and combine with chickpeas and cashew pieces in a large bowl.

- In a small bowl, combine the yogurt, lemon juice, paprika, salt, and curry powder. Mix together with a fork until well combined.

- Toss chickpea mixture with yogurt mixture until well coated.

- Top with scallions and serve in lettuce cups.

CURRIED LENTILS

Curry is a healthy spice that has robust flavor and lends a nice sophistication to this simple-to-prepare meal.

You can use more or less curry to suit the taste of whoever you are cooking for. The coconut milk will "dilute" the intensity of the curry flavor, so taste before you serve and add more if you wish.

To boost the nutrition further, consider adding broccoli, Brussels sprouts, chopped kale or any other healthy green vegetable. Basically, the more greens and the more vegetables you can get in any meal, the better, so use what you have. (Chopping any vegetable in small pieces will allow it to cook faster.)

This easy meal has a nice blend of plant-based protein in the lentils, along with healthy fats and nice complex carbohydrates.

Let us know what variations you come up with.

Ingredients

1 cup dry organic lentils

2 cups organic vegetable broth

4 large organic carrots, diced

Optional: 1 medium organic yellow onion, diced (about 1 cup)

1 tablespoon curry powder

Optional: 2 cloves organic garlic, minced

1 tablespoon organic avocado oil

1 can organic coconut milk

1 cup dry organic quinoa

Method

- Chop the veggies. In a large skillet, heat avocado oil over medium heat.

- Transfer the carrot to the skillet first. Sauté the carrot for about 5 minutes, then add in the garlic and onion. Sauté until tender.

- Mix in the curry powder and add the lentils to the skillet.

- Add broth to the skillet and bring the mixture to a simmer for about 15 to 20 minutes, until the lentils have absorbed the broth and are tender.

- While the lentils are simmering, bring 2 cups of water to a boil and cook the quinoa.

- Mix the coconut milk into the lentil vegetable mixture and allow to simmer until some of the coconut milk has cooked off.

- Serve together on the plate or top the quinoa with the lentil vegetable mixture. You can chop some parsley or green onion to make the dish "prettier" for serving.

MAC 'N CHEESE

Next to mashed potatoes, macaroni and cheese might be the most popular "comfort food" out there. Who doesn't love the carbohydrate-laden, cheesy, warm dish fresh out of the oven with some crunchy breadcrumbs to break up the texture of all the warm, gooey and soft ingredients? It makes you feel good just thinking about it. It may make you feel good mentally perhaps, but physically, is likely another story.

Sorry if I ruined "the moment" but let us be honest. If you are avoiding gluten, dairy, saturated fat or all of the above, traditional mac 'n cheese is just not your friend. That does not mean you can't enjoy a very close substitute, sans gluten, dairy and saturated fat – yay!!

Honestly, my version of the traditional mac 'n cheese is satisfying in all the ways you need it to be – warm, gooey and "cheezy" plus pasta.

Give it a try and tell me how you like it!

Ingredients

1 package gluten-free rice pasta (Jovial brand or better yet, Banza pasta for a high protein, grain-free alternative)

2 cups organic raw cashews

1 ½ cups water

2 tablespoons nutritional yeast

½ teaspoon onion powder

½ teaspoon garlic powder

¼ teaspoon pepper

½ teaspoon salt

¼ teaspoon paprika

3 tablespoons organic vegan butter or healthy oil (tea seed, avocado, etc.)

2 ½ cups Daiya cheese – I used mozzarella, but you could use cheddar.

Method

- Preheat oven to 350°F.

- Soak two cups of cashews covered in water for at least 20 minutes.

- Cook pasta according to package instructions but consider taking it out a minute or two early so as not to overcook. (Italians like their pasta "al dente" and you should cook it this way to prevent mushy pasta once it's done in the oven.) **Note:** this does not apply to the Banza pasta made from chickpeas; follow those package instructions closely.

- Make the cashew cream sauce by placing the soaked cashews, water, nutritional yeast, onion and

- garlic powder, salt and pepper in a blender. Blend on high until very creamy. If it's too thick you can add a little water – the consistency should be that of heavy cream.

- Once the pasta is cooked and drained, place it in a glass dish approximately 9×13".

- Add the vegan butter to the pasta, the Daiya cheese and cashew cream sauce and mix together with a large spoon to evenly coat all the pasta.

- Taste and season with salt and pepper as you see fit. Sprinkle paprika over the top and then cover with the gluten-free breadcrumbs or crackers.

- Bake in 350°F oven for 25 minutes until heated through and slightly crispy on top.

ZUCCHINI CHICKPEA FRITTERS

Zucchini is available all year long for most of us, but summer is an especially fun time to enjoy this veggie. If you plant your own zucchini plants, watching them grow is almost a "Jack and the Beanstalk" moment. They can literally grow inches overnight.

Whether you have a bumper crop or just run over to the grocery store for your zucchini, this healthy veggie (factually it's a fruit but we treat it as a vegetable) provides vitamins C and A plus folate potassium and a nice amount of fiber. It's beneficial for heart health and assists with weight loss.

Fritters are fun to eat but typically contain gluten, dairy and other unhealthy ingredients. These fritters are healthy, filling and have a nice punch of protein from the chickpeas. Plus, they're easy to make.

Ingredients

- 1 large or 2 medium organic zucchinis, grated
- 1 can (13 oz) organic chickpeas rinsed, sautéed for 5 mins in a pan and then mashed with potato masher
- 2 tablespoons organic chickpea flour (I used "garfava" flour, a combination of fava beans and garbanzo beans)
- 2 tablespoons organic almond flour (add more if it feels watery)
- 1 heaped tablespoon nutritional yeast
- salt, to taste
- Optional: Chili powder or paprika, to taste (Just a shake or two is all you need. I used chili powder.)

Optional: 1 clove organic garlic, grated or finely chopped

Optional: ¼ organic red onion, finely chopped

organic avocado oil for pan frying

Method

- Add salt to grated zucchini and toss to coat. Let it rest for 10 minutes and then squeeze the water out of it with your hands. Add to medium sized bowl.

- Add mashed chickpeas, chickpea flour, almond flour, nutritional yeast, chili or paprika, garlic and onion and mix them all together thoroughly.

- Form into patties – they should hold together easily. If too soft, add some more flour.

- Pan fry in avocado oil over medium heat, about 3 to 5 minutes per side. The fritter should be slightly browned.

- Sauce: You can enjoy them as-is or top with any condiment.

SOBA NOODLES WITH ASPARAGUS AND PEAS

This dish has become a family favorite. I always heard soba noodles were difficult to cook, that they tended to stick together, turn into mush, etc. For some reason I haven't experienced any of these problems, but I think the key is to not overcook them, and then thoroughly cool them down with cold water once cooked. (I do spend a few minutes running cold water over the noodles until I can touch them with my fingers and there is no heat remaining in them.)

It's spring as I'm writing this, and asparagus and baby peas are in season. But in the winter I made this with broccoli and in the summer I've used all raw veggies such as red peppers and cherry tomatoes. You can really experiment with what you enjoy. The noodles and sauce stay the same, but the veggies you choose to use are up to you.

The sauce is a little spicy; if you're serving children or adults with a milder palate consider using ¼ teaspoon Cholula and adding more coconut aminos that have a sweet profile.

Please let me know how you enjoy this and any combinations you come up with that you enjoy.

Serves 4

Ingredients

1 package organic 100% buckwheat soba noodles.

1 tablespoon organic avocado oil

Optional: 1 large organic shallot, finely chopped

1 bunch organic asparagus, woody stems removed and cut into ½" pieces

½ bag frozen organic baby peas, or fresh if you can find them in season

5 to 6 organic cremini mushrooms or other mushroom of your choice, sliced thin

1 cup organic red cabbage, sliced thin

Optional: 2 organic green onions, sliced in ¼" pieces

Sauce

2 tablespoons organic almond butter

2 tablespoons organic rice vinegar

2 to 3 teaspoons organic coconut aminos

Optional: 1 teaspoon Cholula hot sauce

Method

- Put a large pot of salted water on high heat. When it is boiling add the soba noodles, stirring to separate the noodles and cook for 8 minutes. (Do not overcook!)

- While the pasta is cooking, heat a sauté pan with avocado oil. Once hot, sauté shallots on medium heat until translucent.

- Add mushrooms and cook on medium-high heat until starting to get some brown color.

- Add the asparagus and peas, reduce heat to medium and sauté until cooked to desire tenderness. (I like to keep the asparagus firm with a little bite to them.) Once cooked, remove from the heat.

- If your pasta is not cooked yet, slice the red cabbage or green onions. If the pasta needs your attention, move this step until later.

- By this time, your pasta should be done. Do not exceed the recommended 8 minutes. Pour the pasta into a sieve and immediately run cold water over it; continue to run cold water for a couple of minutes. Put your clean hands into the pasta and allow the cold water to fully cover all the pasta until there is no warmth left in it. If you do this well your soba noodles will not stick.

- Leave the cooled pasta in the sieve and place all the sauce ingredients into the warm pasta pot. (The warmth helps to combine the ingredients, melting the almond butter.)

- The sauce ingredients are the ratios I used but if you want to add more coconut aminos to cut the "bite" of the vinegar or minimize the spiciness of the Cholula, feel free to make it your own.

- Pour the pasta over the sauce, combine, and then add the veggies (except the green onions), again stirring to combine and coat all ingredients with the sauce.

- Top with sliced green onions and enjoy.

"MEATY" MUSHROOM VEGGIE PATTIES

Who does not love a burger? But we do not necessarily love the problems that come along with eating animal flesh. These meatless burgers are the perfect solution. They are delicious and satisfying and full of "burger joy" without the animal protein.

You can certainly make these burgers from scratch but consider having some extra cooked quinoa and lentils from a meal you have prepared a day or two prior to save yourself some time. Having the quinoa (or rice) and lentils cooked already, make this meal a snap.

You could trade out a different nut for the walnut if you prefer, but otherwise the ingredients listed are best followed exactly.

We like the paleo flour mix because it has no grains in it (therefore less processing), but it does the trick holding the burgers together nicely. Let me know how you like it.

A gluten-free bun is an option if you do okay with refined grains, but otherwise I would enjoy it on a plate topped with the avocado hummus. The tahini dressing can be put on a side salad, or on the bun if you are using one.

(This meal is the creation of Tania, our health coach, so all kudos belong to her.)

Ingredients

<u>Burgers</u>

    1 cup cooked organic quinoa or brown rice

    1 tablespoon organic avocado oil

    Optional: 1 medium organic onion, chopped

    Optional: 2 organic garlic cloves, minced

15 ounces cooked organic lentils

1 cup sautéed organic mushrooms, chopped

1 cup toasted organic walnuts

½ cup Bob's Red Mill Paleo baking flour mix

1 teaspoon dried organic basil

1 teaspoon pink Himalayan sea salt

1 teaspoon ground black pepper

3 tablespoons avocado oil, and more as needed

For burger assembly

bread, your gluten-free choice. (Srsly is a fun brand to try in a loaf or sandwich buns.)

cherry heirloom tomatoes, washed and cut in half lengthwise

salad greens, washed

Avocado hummus

¼ cup organic chickpeas

1 organic avocado, pitted and peeled

⅓ cup packed fresh organic Italian parsley

¼ cup organic avocado oil

Optional: 1 organic garlic clove

1 tablespoon organic apple cider vinegar OR lemon juice

½ teaspoon pink Himalayan sea salt

Optional: ¼ teaspoon red pepper flakes

Tahini salad dressing

½ cup organic tahini

½ cup water

Optional: 1 organic garlic clove

1 tablespoon organic apple cider vinegar OR lemon juice

1 to 1¼ teaspoons pink Himalayan sea salt

½ teaspoon ground black pepper

Optional: ½ teaspoon organic onion powder

Optional: ¼ teaspoon red pepper flakes

Method

- Heat 1 tablespoon of avocado oil in a large pan over medium-high heat, and sauté onions until soft and lightly browned, about 3 to 5 minutes.

- Add garlic and cook another minute or two, stirring frequently to ensure the garlic does not burn. Transfer to a food processor. Reserve skillet for later use.

- Add rice, lentils, walnuts, flour, basil, sea salt, and pepper to the onions in the food processor. Pulse until the walnut pieces are very fine and the mixture comes together. If necessary, transfer the mixture to a large bowl and mix with your hands. Adjust seasoning to taste.

- Form the mixture into eight burger patties with the palms of your hands. You can make your patties thin or a bit thicker depending on preference.

- Heat avocado oil, starting with 1 tablespoon at a time, in the reserved skillet over medium-high heat. Pan fry the patties in batches, adding more oil as needed. Flip the patties and let cook until they are nicely browned on both sides. Remove patties from pan and drain on paper towels.

Avocado hummus

- Combine chickpeas, avocado, parsley, oil, garlic, apple cider vinegar, sea salt, and red pepper flakes (if using) in food processor and puree. Adjust seasoning to taste.

Tahini salad dressing

- In food processor, puree tahini, water, garlic, apple cider vinegar (or lemon juice), sea salt, black pepper, onion powder, and red pepper flakes (if using) until smooth. If too thick, add 1 teaspoon of water as needed. Adjust acidity and flavoring to taste.

Assembling your "meaty" mushroom veggie sandwich/burger or salad

- If using the Srsly bread, cut ½ inch slices and toast. If using sandwich bun, cut in half and toast.

- Spread avocado hummus on each slice of bread. Layer salad greens and sliced tomatoes with veggie patty. Drizzle tahini dressing over top of veggie patty and close sandwich.

Procedure for salad

- In a salad bowl, place 1 to 2 cups of salad greens and top with sliced tomatoes. Top with a couple drizzles of tahini dressing and veggie patty. Serve with a slice of toast topped with avocado hummus on the side.

LENTIL COTTAGE PIE TOPPED WITH SWEET POTATO MASH

This entree is sure to please. It has lentils for protein; healthy onions and garlic for an anti-inflammatory and anti-cancer boost; plus delicious sweet potatoes, rich in antioxidants, vitamins, and minerals.

Did you know sweet potatoes have more potassium than bananas?

This entrée is satisfying AND healthy in addition to being mild in flavor for a younger audience or those who prefer a less robust flavor profile. Personally, I must admit, I like intense flavors in my food, but I realize not everyone is like that, which is why I like this recipe.

Ingredients

Lentil layer

    2 tablespoons organic avocado oil

    Optional: ¼ cup organic shallots, diced

    Optional: 1 tablespoon organic garlic, minced

    ½ pound organic white mushrooms, chopped

    1 cup organic dry green lentils

    2 cups organic carrots, peeled and diced

    Optional: ½ cup organic green onion, chopped

    1 cup frozen organic baby green peas

    2 tablespoons organic parsley, chopped

    ½ teaspoon organic dried thyme

    ¼ teaspoon black pepper

½ teaspoon Himalayan sea salt (taste to see if you would like more)

4 cups organic vegetable stock, plus 4 tablespoons

1 cup organic black lentils

Sweet potato layer

3 medium organic sweet potatoes, peeled and cut into 2″ cubes

Optional: 1 small organic shallot, diced

Optional: 1 organic garlic clove, minced

1 cup unsweetened organic almond milk

½ teaspoon black pepper

¾ teaspoon Himalayan sea salt

½ teaspoon organic dried thyme or oregano

sea salt and black pepper to taste

2 tablespoons arrowroot starch

Method

Lentil layer

- Preheat oven to 400°F.

- In a large pot, heat oil over medium heat until hot.

- Add shallots and sauté about 2 minutes until translucent and lightly golden.

- Add garlic and sauté until fragrant, stirring frequently for about a minute.

- Add green lentils, carrots, green onion, peas, parsley, thyme, black pepper and vegetable stock. Stir with a spoon to combine.

- Bring to a boil, cover, reduce heat to low, and simmer for about 45 minutes to an hour, or until lentils are tender.

- While the green lentils are cooking, in a separate pot, place 1 cup of black lentils in appropriate amount of water (it's typically 2:1 but follow instructions on the bag or box.) Cook on medium until tender. Cooking time is about 30 minutes. Drain when done.

Sweet potato layer

- While the lentil mixture is simmering, place sweet potato in a steamer and cook for about 15 to 20 minutes, until fork tender.

- Remove the sweet potatoes from the steamer and place them in a saucepan over medium-low heat.

- Add shallot and garlic and let sauté for 2 to 3 minutes.

- Add almond milk, pepper, salt, and thyme and combine fully; remove from heat.

- Mash with a vegetable masher until smooth. Season with salt and pepper to taste. Set aside.

- In a small bowl, whisk arrowroot starch and about 4 tablespoons of lentil cooking liquid (if all has evaporated, use vegetable stock) until completely combined.

- Add the arrowroot slurry to the lentils and boil for 2 to 3 minutes, stirring occasionally, until the sauce thickens. Stir in cooked black lentils. Season with salt and pepper to taste.

- Transfer lentil filling into a 9×9″ or 9×13″ glass baking dish. (The larger dish will make the pie less deep, which I think is preferable.) Using a clean spoon, scoop and spread sweet potato mash on top of the cooked lentil mixture, creating a thin layer that completely covers the lentils.

- Place on the middle oven rack and cook for about 30 minutes until the lentil mixture is bubbling and mashed sweet potatoes are slightly crispy. Serve hot.

MAPLE ROASTED BRUSSELS SPROUTS
WITH TOASTED PECANS

Brussels sprouts are a very healthy vegetable. They are part of the cruciferous family along with kale, arugula, and broccoli. Brussels sprouts are miniature cabbages that, when prepared correctly, are delicious.

Personally, I remember having a strong dislike for them as a child. My mother was a great cook but apparently no one told her about the trick of roasting Brussels sprouts. Hers were boiled and very unappealing to look at, not to mention eat.

I always try to include the healthiest foods in my diet, so I well remember the day I purchased Brussels sprouts, deciding that I would find a way to enjoy them. We actually have a couple of recipes on our site for them, but they do tend to pair great with nuts, especially creamy pecans.

This particular recipe includes maple syrup because it's the holiday season and we are trying to offer up some sweetness while maintaining the health quotient of recipes. But you can definitely (preferably) leave out or use less maple syrup and you will still have a delicious dish.

Ingredients

1 ½ pounds organic Brussels sprouts

¼ cup organic avocado oil

¾ teaspoon Himalayan sea salt

¼ teaspoon black pepper

2 tablespoons 100% pure organic maple syrup

½ cup coarsely chopped toasted organic pecans

Method

- Preheat oven to 375°F.

- Prepare Brussels sprouts: remove any yellow or brown outer leaves, cut off the stems, and cut in half. Rinse and dry.

- In a large bowl, toss the sprouts in oil, salt, and pepper. Once all the sprouts are coated in oil, arrange them in a 9×13″ baking sheet.

- Roast for 15 minutes, then stir sprouts around with a spatula to even out the browning. Continue to roast for an additional 25 to 30 minutes.

- Stir the sprouts again, and drizzle maple syrup over the top.

- Roast the sprouts for a final 10 to 15 minutes or until fork tender (about 40 to 45 minutes total roasting time).

<u>To toast pecans</u>

- Preheat oven to 350°F.

- Place the pecans in one layer on a rimmed baking sheet. Roast for 8 to 10 minutes, or until lightly browned and fragrant. Keep checking on them because nuts can burn quickly.

- Toss the roasted sprouts with pecans and serve warm.

SOBA NOODLE VEGETABLE SALAD

If you are trying to avoid refined carbohydrates, you may think pasta salad is a thing of the past. It does not need to be. This salad is incredibly filling AND healthy, utilizing buckwheat noodles, a fun and flavorful dressing, and uber-healthy veggies.

Do not let the name fool you: buckwheat is completely gluten-free. In fact, buckwheat is a seed, not a grain, despite that confusing "wheat" word in its name. Therefore, this recipe is grain-free and refined carbohydrate free.

Buckwheat is a resistant starch, meaning it tends to make its way down into your colon and feed your healthy gut bacteria, something you definitely want. For more on resistant starch read this blog, "Starch you don't have to resist" on my website: *www.RootCauseMedicalClinics.com.*

Buckwheat is good for your heart through its ability to lower cholesterol and blood pressure; it's an excellent source of fiber, which makes it good in preventing many diseases including cancer; it reduces your risk of diabetes, and it is high in antioxidants, vitamins and minerals.

Make sure when you buy buckwheat noodles, they are 100% buckwheat and thereby gluten-free. Some noodles in the market mix wheat with the buckwheat – please avoid those.

When cooking buckwheat noodles avoid salting the water, do not overcook (follow package directions), and once drained, immediately put them in a bowl of very cold water. Stir the noodles around with your hands in the cold water to rinse off their starch for just a minute or so and then re-drain. This procedure will prevent them from sticking together.

Any vegetable you want to add is fine, but as always, I suggest the ones that provide the best nutrition: those of the cruciferous and allium families. They are the best anti-cancer, anti-inflammatory vegetables you can eat.

The sauce can be made more or less spicy depending on whom you are feeding – play with it and feel free to send me the combination you enjoy most. (See our web site for your coconut aminos, date syrup and gluten-free Tamari.)

Please let me know how you enjoy this and what varieties you come up with.

Servings: 2

Ingredients

½ package of buckwheat noodles, cooked, drained and rinsed in cold water

½ organic red pepper OR zucchini, sliced thinly

2 organic green onions cut into ¼ to ½" rounds

2 cups organic purple cabbage, sliced thinly or chopped

1 small organic carrot, grated

1 to 2 tablespoons organic cilantro chopped

Sauce

1 scant tablespoon organic almond butter

1 scant tablespoon organic avocado oil

1 teaspoon organic gluten-free Tamari

2 teaspoons organic coconut aminos

Optional: 2 teaspoons organic lemon juice

2 pinches organic ginger powder

¼ teaspoon organic date syrup (option: maple syrup, but date is so much healthier)

Optional (for the "adult palate): ½ teaspoon red pepper flakes

Method

- Bring a pot of water to the boil. (Do not add salt to the water.) Add buckwheat noodles and cook about 8 minutes, according to package directions. (Do not overcook!)

- While the noodles are cooking, chop and grate your veggies.

- Drain the noodles and then immerse in a bowl of very cold water. Stir noodles around with your hands for a minute or two – this will remove excess starch and prevent them from sticking together. Re-drain the noodles.

- Mix up the sauce by placing all ingredients into a bowl and whisking together with a fork. Taste and add more lemon juice (to lighten and brighten the flavor) or coconut aminos (to lightly sweeten the dish) as needed.

- You can combine the dry ingredients in advance and add the sauce later when you are ready to eat.

GRILLED TERIYAKI TOFU

It is important you get enough healthy protein on a plant-based (or predominantly plant-based) diet. Have you heard you should avoid soy? Get the truth about soy here on my blog: "Should you eat soy or avoid it?"

This recipe is fun to bring to a grilling party, or simply to enjoy at home. It could not be simpler, yet it is delicious, packs a nice plant-based protein "punch," and is very satisfying.

Serve it with a big healthy salad and black rice (that was how I served it to my family, and I cooked black beluga lentils with the rice.)

Tip: Throw some lentils, green, black or red into your rice cooker to amp up the protein content of your rice.

This recipe is fast, healthy and delicious. Let me know how you enjoy it!

Servings: 4

Ingredients

- 1 package extra firm organic tofu
- 3 to 6 tablespoons organic teriyaki coconut aminos for marinating and topping once cooked
- 1 tablespoon avocado oil for the grill pan

Method

- Remove the tofu from the water it comes in. Each 8-ounce piece can be cut in quarters, about ½ inch thick. Pat each piece in paper towels to remove the excess water. Push down a little to remove the water.

- Place 3 to 4 pieces into a dinner plate and add about 2 tablespoons of the Teriyaki coconut aminos. (You will need two dinner plates to marinate enough for 4 people.)

- Flip the pieces every 5 minutes or so until they are fully marinated – about 15 minutes total. (If they sit in the marinade longer it is completely fine.)

- Once they are marinated, heat the grill pan on medium high and add the oil. Once the pan is hot, place the tofu onto the heated surface and grill for about 3 minutes. The tofu should sizzle, and when you flip it you'll see nice grill marks.

- Cook for another 3 minutes and serve with a salad, other veggies, etc.

- You can top with more Teriyaki sauce if you desire.

MUSHROOM STROGANOFF

I used to love mushroom stroganoff. Of course, I loved anything that involved gluten and dairy (can you guess what foods I'm sensitive to? LOL!) Pasta was a particularly favored version of gluten. Therefore, mushroom stroganoff definitely fit all the categories: noodles covered in creamy, mushroom goodness with a dollop of sour cream, as if it needed more dairy!

Once you change your diet as radically as I changed mine, there are certain foods and dishes you feel you will never see again. I don't know why I never thought to create my own version, but recently when my husband said he was craving cream of mushroom soup, I realized it would be pretty easy to make a plant-based version. It came out great (which reminds me, I need to put up that recipe as well.)

While in the midst of creating the recipe, the "soup" was very thick. Before I thinned it out, I tasted it and the flavor reminded me of my old favorite: mushroom stroganoff. I was committed to the soup at that moment, but I decided that I would take the foundation of the soup and see if I could recreate stroganoff.

My family loved it and I hope you will too. The extra sour cream that is part of traditional stroganoff was created through a synthesis of about three or four different recipes I viewed online, plus my own input. That recipe is just below.

Let me know how you enjoy this and if you come up with any variations you enjoy.

Ingredients

1 box gluten-free noodles or rotini pasta (my favorite is Banza pasta because it is grain-free, but Jovial pasta is another alternative for a rice-based pasta. I would not use a spaghetti; the sauce would be too heavy for it.)

Optional: 1 large or 2 small organic shallots, finely minced

Optional: 2 cloves organic garlic, minced

3 cups of chopped organic crimini mushrooms (or your favorite organic mushrooms)

1 tablespoon organic avocado oil

Optional: 2 tablespoons white wine (all the alcohol gets cooked off; it just adds some flavor to the mushrooms)

¼ teaspoon of organic oregano

¾ teaspoon of organic thyme

1 box (32 oz) organic vegetable broth (you may not use the full amount)

1 cup organic raw cashews

Salt and pepper to taste

vegan sour cream (see recipe on my website: *www. RootCauseMedicalClinics.com)*

Method

- Put a large pot of water on to boil. Add about 2 tablespoons of salt to the water.
- While waiting for the water to boil, chop your mushrooms, shallots and garlic.

- Put the oil in a large sauté pan and heat on medium. Once warm, add the shallots and cook about 3 minutes, until softened.

- Raise the heat to medium-high and add the mushrooms. (Heat needs to be fairly high under mushrooms to pull the water out from them and brown them.)

- Add the herbs, plus the white wine (if you are using it), at this point.

- Your water should be boiling; add the pasta and make sure you do not overcook it.

- Once the mushrooms have been cooking about 4 minutes and are getting browned, add the garlic for an additional minute or two. Be careful not to burn the garlic. If anything is starting to get too brown, use a splash of vegetable broth to prevent any burning or sticking.

- Take ¾ of the cooked mushrooms and place in a high-speed blender with 2 cups of the vegetable broth and the cashews. The broth is not heated, so no worries about blending a hot liquid.

- Blend on high, adding more veggie broth as needed until smooth and the desired thickness. The sauce should be fairly thick and very creamy.

- Add salt and pepper to taste.

- Place the sauce back into the original sauté pan to heat.

- The pasta should be done about this time. Strain it and add it to the heated sauce.

- Top with a dollop of dairy-free sour cream and serve immediately.

PAD THAI

Do you love pad thai? My family does. Traditionally it is a Thai noodle dish that is fried and contains eggs and a fish sauce. The only thing that "works" about the traditional pad thai is that it's gluten-free. Initially when we discovered a problem with gluten, anything naturally gluten-free that could be found in a restaurant was very exciting. Pad thai was one such dish.

Of course, time marched on and we became dairy-free (Pad thai still fit the bill) and then plant-based. It was this latter evolution of our diet that caused the problem: the fish sauce was no longer going to work.

I began to be concerned about the status of the tofu (it was doubtful restaurants were serving organic and therefore GMO-free), and then there was the frying. What kind of oils were they using? Typically, the answer was canola or peanut, neither of which was healthy.

One day I declared to my family that I thought I could make a vegan version. I was met with some doubtful looks. I persevered and with the help of some on-line inspiration, arrived at the recipe below.

Full disclosure: this recipe is "fussy". By that I mean there are a lot of ingredients. There is nothing difficult in the preparation, it's just time consuming to measure out the long list of ingredients. If you have a friend or family member who will join you in the prep process, it becomes easy and of course more fun!

Mung bean sprouts are a traditional ingredient in pad thai. I frequently have trouble finding them, so I substitute cooked sprouted mung beans, which are very good for you, make the meal heartier and have good protein and nice anti-cancer properties.

Unlike most of the meals I prepare there is nothing truly "green" in this one, unless you count the green onions. Therefore, I like the addition of the cooked mung beans for their health benefits. (Of course, I've been known to quietly finely chop some organic kale and throw it in, but don't tell anyone!)

Serves 4

Ingredients

- 8 ounces pad thai rice noodles
- 6 tablespoons organic smooth almond butter
- 1 tablespoon tamarind paste
- 2 teaspoons avocado oil, divided
- 5 tablespoons organic tamari (gluten-free), divided into 3 tablespoons and 2 tablespoons
- 2 tablespoons maple syrup
- Optional: 1 ½ tablespoons sriracha, to taste
- Optional: ⅓ cup organic lemon (or lime) juice
- ½ cup water
- 1 tablespoon avocado oil
- Optional: 1 clove garlic, minced
- One bag of Quorn Chik'n Tenders or 14 ounce block of extra firm organic tofu, drained
- 1 tablespoon grated ginger
- 2 large organic carrots, cut into thin strips
- Optional: 4 organic green onions, halved lengthwise and cut into ½" pieces

1 cup cooked sprouted mung beans (I use TruRoots variety: ¾ cup dried yields about 1 cup cooked) OR 1 cup mung bean sprouts

½ cup cilantro or parsley, chopped

¼ cup organic peanuts, chopped

Optional: Lemon slices, for garnish

Method

- Cook the pad thai noodles according to the package instructions. Rinse with cold water until no longer warm, then toss them with a teaspoon of avocado oil to prevent sticking.

- Cook the sprouted mung beans according to package directions to make 1 ½ cups cooked. Drain and set aside. (You can omit this step if you are using actual mung bean sprouts.)

- Whisk or blend together the almond butter, tamarind paste, the remaining teaspoon of avocado oil, 3 tablespoons of tamari, maple syrup, sriracha, lemon juice, and water. Set aside.

- Taste the sauce. If it is too spicy for you, consider adding more lemon juice, tamari and/or water, depending on your taste.

- Heat the avocado oil in a large skillet over medium high heat. Add the Quorn (or tofu) and cook until it's browning on each side (8 to 10 minutes), splashing it as you go with the remaining tablespoon or two of tamari. Set Quorn (tofu) aside in a bowl and reduce heat on your skillet to medium.

- Add the garlic and ginger to the skillet (and a little extra oil if needed). Cook until the garlic is fragrant, 1 to 2 minutes. Add the carrots and onions and cook until the carrots are softened but still crisp, about 3 minutes.

- Add the noodles to the bowl with the Quorn and pour a cup of the sauce over them and stir to coat the noodles.

- Now pour the noodles and Quorn into the skillet with the veggies, add the cooked mung beans if you are using and stir fry the noodles until they're warm. Add more sauce as you go along to ensure everything is well coated.

- If you are using mung bean sprouts, stir them in now to warm them.

- Divide the noodles onto four plates. Sprinkle with cilantro (or parsley) and peanuts and garnish with lime (or lemon). Serve.

NUTTY GREEN RICE

I am always looking for ways to elevate to a healthier status the carb-rich dishes that patients desire. This easy, tasty dish does just that. If you have never tried Banza rice, it is a grain-free alternative made from garbanzo beans. I recommend you try it.

If you are sticking with traditional rice, first you begin with a healthy version: black rice is the best, with brown rice next in line. Try to stay away from the white, highly refined rice. It is important to place rice in a sieve and rinse it very well under cold water to remove the excess starch before cooking it.

Rice takes a while to cook, therefore it gives you time to see what's lurking in the vegetable drawer. I've given some suggestions below (in the list of ingredients), but the idea is to add a nice variety of healthy veggies (raw, or lightly steamed/sautéed) to amp up the health value of this meal.

Originally this dish was designed as a room temperature recipe to be served with raw vegetables, more appropriate when the weather is warmer. However, I have also enjoyed it warm with lightly steamed or sautéed vegetables and either way is delicious.

What's fun is to add what you have on hand, making the variety of this dish almost endless.

Beans are something that protect against disease, especially cancer, and extend life expectancy, so any excuse to add beans to a meal is a great idea. This particular dish is very well suited to an addition of healthy beans, either warm or cold.

Let me know what delicious combinations you come up with.

Enjoy!

Ingredients

1 cup organic brown basmati or black rice, well rinsed. A grain-free alternative is Banza rice, which cooks up fast and is made from garbanzo beans.

2 cups water

¼ to ½ teaspoon salt

½ cup organic almonds

1 bunch organic parsley

1 clove garlic

1 ½ tablespoons lemon juice, or substitute

Optional: 1 tablespoon rice wine vinegar

1 ½ tablespoons organic olive oil

½ organic cucumber, diced

salt and pepper to taste

Optional: chopped olives, organic red or yellow pepper, chopped green onion and/or red cabbage can all be added to bring more nutrition into this dish, not to mention color! Another option is rinsed cooked beans such as black beans, garbanzo beans or cannellini.

Method

- Add water and rice into rice cooker. When cooked, add salt and serve warm or allow to cool. (If using the Banza rice it is easy and fast on the stovetop.)

- While rice is cooking, blend almonds, parsley, garlic, and oil in a food processor.

- Stir in nut mixture and add salt and pepper to taste.

- Place cucumber and/or other cold or lightly cooked vegetables and beans over top of the rice and combine.

FALL VEGETABLE RISOTTO

There are many ways to prepare rice, but this hearty dish is a favorite. It's pretty to look at while including healthy vegetables that boost the antioxidant, anti-cancer properties.

Risotto takes a little time to prepare but it is in no way difficult.

Many variations exist for this recipe, not the least of which is utilizing your favorite vegetables or whatever you have on hand. You also do not need to use risotto rice. A healthier version that takes about the same length of time is brown rice. It is equally "chewy" and substantial but has a higher nutrient value.

This recipe calls for butternut squash, broccoli and kale. You can easily substitute other vegetables such as sweet potatoes, Brussels sprouts and spinach. Think of color variety when making this dish, not only so that it looks attractive, but also to provide a variety of healthy nutrients.

Try to include cruciferous vegetables whenever you can as they are some of the healthiest. The cruciferous family includes kale, collard greens, broccoli, cauliflower, Brussels sprouts and more!

Please let me know how you enjoy this and what delicious varieties you come up with!

(For the inspiration of this recipe, I would like to thank fooduzzi. com, a fellow Italian with a mind towards making the classics healthy!)

Ingredients

3 tablespoons organic avocado oil

2 cups organic butternut squash, diced into bite-size chunks

2 cups organic broccoli florets, bite-sized but not too small or they'll burn

1 box (32 oz) organic vegetable stock (about 4 cups)

Optional: ½ organic yellow onion, diced

Optional: 1 to 2 cloves garlic, minced

¾ cup brown rice or risotto rice

2 to 4 tablespoon Daiya or Myokos cheese, mozzarella style

1 tablespoon nutritional yeast

pinch of red pepper flakes or a pinch of freshly-ground nutmeg (optional)

2 handfuls finely chopped organic kale

some Himalayan sea salt and pepper to taste

Method

- Preheat the oven to 425°F. Line a baking sheet with parchment paper.

- Add diced butternut squash and broccoli to the lined baking sheet. Drizzle with 1 tablespoon avocado oil, season with salt and pepper and toss with your hands to ensure vegetables are well coated.

- Place in the oven until the squash is fork-tender, 20 to 25 minutes. **Note:** Keep an eye on the broccoli to ensure it does not get overcooked. You may need to remove it before the squash is fully done.

- While the vegetables are roasting, add vegetable stock to a medium saucepan and heat until just about to boil. Reduce to a simmer.

- Once the stock is simmering, start making your risotto. Heat a medium-sized skillet over medium-low heat.

- Add 1 tablespoon avocado oil and the diced onion. Season with salt and pepper, and sauté until onion is translucent, about 5 minutes. Add minced garlic and stir to combine.

- Reduce the heat to low. Add risotto rice and stir to coat in the avocado oil.

- Toast the rice for a minute or two, then add 1 cup of simmering stock. Season with salt and pepper to taste, then stir. The key to good risotto is almost constant stirring. It develops the starch, lending to the creaminess of classic risotto.

- When the stock has been almost completely absorbed, add another cup of stock, continuing to stir. Continue to repeat the process until rice is "al dente" (soft with a little chewiness to it), anywhere from 30 to 45 minutes. You may not need all of the stock, depending on the type of rice you choose.

- Add Daiya cheese (if using) and nutritional yeast to the mixture at the end of cooking. Add red pepper flakes or nutmeg if desired.

- About 5 minutes before your risotto is finished cooking (about the half-hour mark into preparation), add 1 tablespoon avocado oil, kale, salt, and pepper to a skillet. Sauté until kale is tender and bright green, about 3 minutes.

- Add butternut squash, broccoli, and kale to the risotto and mix well. Top with additional Daiya cheese if using and/or freshly cracked pepper.

CAULIFLOWER CURRY

Sometimes you just do not have the time or energy to fix a meal. I understand. I cook dinner for my family six days a week and while I enjoy it most of the time, there are those occasional evenings where I wish someone was at home cooking for me.

The good news is…this recipe! The only secret is a cauliflower, a jar of curry sauce and a box/can of beans.

A nice feature of cauliflower is that it easily keeps in the refrigerator for well over a week. The trick is to have one on hand or make a quick grocery store run. The simmer sauce and beans keep "forever" so that is easy too.

Despite the need to hurry, you can still be committed to feeding yourself and family well. Look no further than this ridiculously fast, easy and very healthy vegan meal.

You could also substitute another vegetable such as broccoli or Brussels sprouts for the cauliflower, and a substitute for garbanzo beans could be cannelini or your favorite white bean.

The Maya Kaimal company makes a variety of jarred sauces. The particular one I recommend is gluten-free, dairy-free and delicious.

Give this a try when you are too tired or rushed to spend more than 20 minutes in the kitchen. Your family will still think you were cooking for hours because the meal has such a sophisticated flavor profile. If the sauce is too spicy for some members of your family, you can easily "dilute" it with coconut milk or cream.

Serves 3 to 4

Ingredients

1 jar (12.5 oz) Maya Kaimal Indian Simmer Sauce, Madras Curry

1 organic cauliflower, cut into bite-size florets

1 can or box of organic garbanzo beans, drained and rinsed

organic whole fat coconut milk or cashew cream sauce

Optional: 1 to 2 cups cooked organic brown rice

Method

- If you need to prepare rice, start with that. (Rice is not mandatory and if you're avoiding grains, this dish holds up on its own without it.) As an alternative, try Banza rice which is made from garbanzo beans.

- Cut the cauliflower into bite-size florets and steam for 3 minutes.

- Open the can or box of beans and drain and rinse thoroughly.

- Open the jar of simmer sauce and pour the entire contents into a large saucepan on medium heat.

- If spice can bother your stomach, start with half the jar plus the coconut cream.

- Once the cauliflower is steamed, add it directly into the sauce along with the beans and warm through.

- If you need to make it less spicy you can add some coconut or cashew cream to temper the spice. (This is also a good way to add some healthy fat to the meal.)

- Serve over the rice or alone with a salad.

SWEET POTATO ALFREDO PASTA

Pasta alfredo was my favorite in my gluten- and dairy-eating days. I always felt terrible after eating it, but I wasn't really aware enough in those days to make the association. Leaving gluten and dairy behind, I felt my alfredo days were behind me.

This creamy, luscious, and satisfying alfredo pasta has no dairy, gluten, or grains. Plus, it's high in protein, courtesy of the bean-based pasta.

It boasts healthy sweet potatoes, is rich in antioxidants, plus it is filling and truly delicious.

It is fast and easy to make, so coming home a little late won't prevent you from enjoying this fun meal.

Ingredients

1 box Banza pasta, elbow shape or penne

1 steamed or boiled medium to large organic sweet potato

½ cup organic almond milk, unsweetened

½ cup organic veggie broth

2 teaspoons organic oregano

Optional: 1 teaspoon organic garlic powder

½ teaspoon Himalayan sea salt

1 tablespoon organic extra-virgin cold pressed olive oil

1 tablespoon organic lemon juice

Method

- Bring the water to a boil for the pasta and sweet potato separately. Salt the pasta water.

- Chop potato into ½" cubes.

- Cook pasta according to package instructions. Drain in a colander when done.

- Steam or boil potato for 15 to 20 minutes, or until tender when pierced with a fork.

- Take remaining ingredients, add to a medium bowl, and mix together with a whisk until fully combined.

- Drain cooked potato and add to bowl, stirring to combined. Add strained pasta and stir to combine all ingredients.

- Serve and enjoy!

HIGH PROTEIN PASTA WITH "CREAM" SAUCE

I love pasta – always have. Of course, it didn't love me, considering I was gluten sensitive, but who knew? I grew up with an Italian father and Italian was my "go to" food choice.

One of my favorite pasta dishes was fettucine alfredo – my dad's name was "Alfred" so we used to joke about that. One day I discovered a pink sauce; it was basically alfredo sauce with a dollop of marinara sauce to make it pink. It was pretty to look at, and pretty darn delicious to eat.

Of course, I felt terrible most of the time since I basically "lived" on gluten and dairy – two foods I completely don't tolerate. Sound familiar? Perhaps you too have discovered gluten and dairy to not be your friends. If so, you are in very good company and our site can now be your new friend – not a single recipe contains either ingredient! :-))

I am always trying to improve the health quotient of my recipes. While I am a huge pasta fan, as previously stated, I am not a big fan of refined grains. So, while rice pasta is "okay", it is not ideal and I'm always going for ideal!

Enter garbanzo bean pasta! I was suspicious when my daughter brought it home. I'll admit to being a pasta snob and while I have tried less refined products made with quinoa, black beans and other ingredients, I hadn't found one I liked. My skepticism made this pasta an even better surprise – I loved it.

Some hints about the pasta – do not undercook it. If you are Italian like me, or just like to cook, you will know that pasta should be cooked "al dente" – which means it has a little "tooth" or firmness to it. This pasta is different. You want to cook it fully, which takes about 7 to 9 minutes.

It is dense, which makes it filling. Of course, it is loaded with protein, unlike typical pasta, so you will find you can't eat as much as you typically might. But that is one of the things I love about it – around 20 grams of protein, filling and NO refined grains.

Now the fun part is the sauce. If you are in a rush there's nothing wrong with opening a jar of your favorite organic pasta sauce, as long as the ingredients are healthy. But don't you want to try a luscious creamy "pink" sauce? Yum!

The recipe below is a small variation on my classic cashew cream sauce, with the pink coming from roasted red peppers. If you dislike red peppers you could always make the basic sauce and add some pasta sauce to turn it pink – there are endless variations.

And, of course, I encourage you to add some sautéed (or lightly steamed) vegetables to your pasta or serve it with a large salad.

I hope you enjoy this pasta as much as I do. A patient recently told me about a black bean pasta she enjoys. If you have a specific brand you have tried and liked, let me know.

Ingredients

- 1 box Banza pasta (rotini is what I used, but choose whatever shape you like)
- 1 ½ cups of organic cashews (soaked for at least 15 minutes, longer is fine)
- 1 cup of filtered water
- Optional: ¼ teaspoon of garlic powder
- Optional: ¼ teaspoon of onion powder

1 tablespoon of nutritional yeast

1 tablespoon of organic lemon juice

1 organic whole roasted red pepper (Jarred is fine. You can start with less if you like.)

salt to taste

Method

- Soak cashews.

- Bring salted water to a boil. Add the pasta to the water and stir well to ensure none stick to the bottom. In about 5 minutes stir it again.

- While the pasta is cooking, drain the cashews and put them into a high-speed blender.

- Add the water, garlic powder, onion powder, nutritional yeast, lemon juice, red pepper. Blend until very smooth.

- Taste the sauce and decide what it needs. More lemon? If you like the red pepper flavor, consider adding another one. If you like it "cheesier" then consider an extra tablespoon of nutritional yeast. Salt can be added now as well.

- Make sure the pasta is fully cooked and then drain it.

- Pour over pasta and enjoy!

TEN-VEGETABLE SOUP WITH TEMPEH

Servings: 4

Ingredients

2 tablespoons extra-virgin olive oil

3 cups chopped green cabbage, quartered

1 cup cauliflower florets, 1″ pieces

Optional: 1 medium leek, sliced (use the white part plus 1″ of the light green part)

Optional: 1 small onion, chopped

1 medium carrot, chopped

1 medium celery stalk, chopped

Optional: 1 can (14.5 oz) diced tomatoes (no salt added)

4 cups low-sodium vegetable broth

1 medium yellow-fleshed potato, diced

¼ cup chopped flat-leaf parsley, fresh

1 tablespoon dried thyme

1 ½ cups packed Swiss chard or spinach, cut crosswise into ½″ strips

2 cups organic tempeh, gluten-free

½ teaspoon sea salt

¼ teaspoon freshly ground pepper

Optional: a pinch of red pepper flakes or cayenne

Method

- Using a large Dutch oven or heavy soup pot with tight-fitting cover, heat oil over medium heat.

- Add cabbage, cauliflower, leek, onion, carrot, and celery. Stirring occasionally, cook vegetables until cabbage is limp and onion translucent (about 4 to 5 minutes). Cover, reduce heat to low, and cook about 8 minutes (until vegetables release their juices).

- Add tomatoes (with the liquid), broth, potato, parsley and thyme. Increase heat to medium-high until liquid boils. Cover, reduce heat, and simmer soup for 10 minutes.

- Add Swiss chard and tempeh, and simmer for 10 minutes. Season soup with sea salt and pepper (and red pepper flakes, if desired). Let sit for 15 minutes before serving.

- Tips: If desired, refrigerate for up to four days, reheating in covered pot over medium heat. Or divide cooled soup among re-sealable freezer bags and freeze. (This soup keeps in the freezer for up to two months.)

GARLIC MASHED CAULIFLOWER

Servings: 4

Ingredients

1 medium head organic cauliflower

2 tablespoons virgin organic coconut oil

3 tablespoons canned organic coconut milk

¼ teaspoon sea salt

Optional: 1 clove fresh garlic, or 1 teaspoon garlic powder
(Option: Asafoetida can be used as an alternative to
garlic.)

¼ teaspoon black pepper

Method

- Cut cauliflower into 4 to 6 pieces and steam until cooked
  but not overdone.

- Place in food processor with remaining ingredients,
  including herbs of your choice, and blend until
  cauliflower is the consistency of mashed potatoes. Serve
  immediately.

SALMON WITH ROASTED CHERRIES

Servings: 4

Ingredients

¾ pound cherries, pitted & halved (about 3 cups)

3 tablespoons fresh lemon juice, divided

Optional: 1 tablespoon maple syrup or honey

2 teaspoons chopped fresh thyme

1 pound (4 fillets) wild caught Pacific salmon (avoid Atlantic or farm-raised salmon)

Method

- Prepare the cherries by pitting and halving. Place in medium to large bowl. Toss with 1 tablespoon lemon juice, sweetener, and fresh thyme.

- Arrange salmon skin-side down on a large parchment-lined baking sheet.

- Spread cherry mixture over salmon. Broil salmon until just cooked through, and cherries are caramelized, 5–7 minutes.

- Transfer to plates, drizzle with remaining 2 tablespoons lemon juice.

- Tips: This is great served over rice or quinoa or a bed of fresh spinach

DESSERTS

FRESH BERRIES WITH COCONUT MANGO CREAM

Servings: 4

Ingredients

⅔ cup organic coconut milk, canned

1⅓ cup organic diced frozen mango (do not defrost)

1 teaspoon vanilla

2 cups fresh organic blueberries, raspberries, or blackberries

Method

- In a blender, add coconut milk and frozen mango. Blend on high until smooth.

- Add vanilla and blend again for several seconds.

- Evenly divide berries among four dishes. Top with coconut cream.

- Tips: For a variation, add ⅓ cup frozen raspberries to the coconut milk and mango in the first step. The pink color is beautiful on top of the berries.

APPLE CRISP

When apples are in season, it is fun to enjoy this healthy fruit. (Remember to only consume the organic varieties; apples tend to be heavily sprayed with pesticides, putting them on the "Dirty Dozen" list of fruits and veggies to be avoided.)

My husband loves "crisps" but when you are avoiding gluten and dairy and oats, not to mention refined sugar, the challenge can seem insurmountable. He was extremely happy with this dairy-free apple crisp recipe that has no grains and no refined sugar. I hope you enjoy it too!

Ingredients

5 organic Fuji or Granny Smith apples, cored and sliced

½ cup of coconut sugar or granulated monk fruit

½ teaspoon of cinnamon

¼ teaspoon of organic vanilla

1 ¾ cup of Dr. Vikki's Granola (the recipe is in this chapter)

1 cup filtered water

Method

- Place 1 cup of filtered water and sliced apples in a medium saucepan.

- Add ¼ cup of coconut sugar, ½ teaspoon of cinnamon and ¼ teaspoon of vanilla to the apple mixture and cook on medium heat for 5 to 10 minutes or until apples have begun to soften.

- Once cooked, add the apples along with all the liquid to a medium size glass dish.

- Top with Dr. Vikki's Granola and sprinkle ¼ cup of coconut sugar or honey on top.

- Bake in a 350°F oven for about 20 minutes or until granola is golden. Serve by itself or with coconut ice cream or coconut whipped cream.

FUDGY BROWNIES

Healthy Brownies with a Twist

The first time I made these brownies I was not yet completely plant-based in my diet. I thought I was doing well with gluten-free and dairy-free and minimal sugar! My children say one day all I will eat is dirt and sticks, but I think they're exaggerating… I mean, where are the nutrients??

I like to keep desserts to a minimum, but sometimes you just want something sweet while still maintaining your healthy diet. After several tries, I mastered how to make these fudgy and rich without the eggs, so if you're avoiding eggs, the plant-based version is noted below, making it a super healthy version of a ridiculously fudgy, chocolatey, decadent brownie.

The secret ingredient really boosts the health aspect, not to mention packing a protein punch. These are very fast to whip up and your family and friends will likely never guess the secret. I remember having a guessing game at a dinner party I hosted. There were a lot of interesting guesses as to what the secret ingredient might be, but no one actually got it right. When I told them, they were pretty shocked!

I do recommend using cacao vs. cocoa powder – small spelling difference, big health difference! The brownies will not be super sweet due to the use of healthier coconut or date sugar, but once again, much healthier. You can use pecans if you prefer them to walnuts: both nuts have great anti-cancer properties.

Let me know how you enjoy these! (And see if your guests can figure out the secret ingredient!)

Ingredients

1 can or box (~ 15 oz) organic black beans, rinsed well

3 organic eggs OR for a plant-based recipe substitute the
following (one option for each of the 3 eggs, plus
additional options follow)

*"Flax egg" (helpful in leavening, makes it rise, plus binding):
combine 1 tablespoon organic ground flax with 3 tablespoons
warm water. Combine and let sit for 10 minutes until thick.*

*¼ cup ripe avocado, mashed (good for binding.) Must be ripe but
not over-ripe – an "off" flavor will ruin your brownies.*

*Combine 1 teaspoon baking soda with 1 tablespoon apple cider
vinegar (a good leavening agent) Once it's done "fizzing,"
add to wet ingredients.*

Additional egg substitute options:

- *Arrowroot powder (good for binding.) Mix 2 tablespoons of
preferred starch with 3 tablespoons water.*

- *Nut butter (good for binding.) The creamy texture works well
to bind cookies, pancakes, and brownies. Use 3 tablespoon
organic creamy nut butter to replace one egg.*

- *Chia egg (helps in leavening and binding.) Prepared exactly the
same as a flax egg above, just substitute ground chia.*

- *Baking powder (leavening agent.) If the recipe doesn't already
call for baking powder, replace one egg by mixing 2
tablespoons of water with 1 tablespoon oil of choice plus two
tablespoons of baking powder.*

- *Mashed banana (binding agent.) Take half an organic banana and mash it well to replace an egg. It works well with cookies, pancakes and brownie. Much like the avocado option, ensure your banana is nicely ripe but not over ripe such that it will impart an odd flavor.*

- *Applesauce (for moisture.) Use ¼ cup unsweetened organic applesauce to replace 1 egg.*

- *Silken tofu (for moisture.) Use ¼ cup organic silken tofu to replace one egg.*

3 tablespoons of avocado oil or other healthy oil such as refined coconut or almond

¾ cups organic coconut or date sugar

¼ cup organic cacao powder

1 teaspoon pure vanilla

½ teaspoon baking powder

⅛ teaspoon Himalayan sea salt

½ cup high quality dark chocolate chips, dairy and soy free. (Option, but they do make it more decadent: You can also make your own sugar-free chocolate by following the recipe on my website: *www.RootCauseMedicalClinics.com.* Lily's chocolate chips are another option for purchase; they are sweetened with stevia.)

½ cup organic raw walnuts, chopped

Method

- Preheat oven to 350°F.

- Grease a glass 8x8" pan with the oil of your choice.

- Mash the beans with a potato masher or blend them in a blender with the oil to break them up.

- Take all the rest of the ingredients, except the chocolate chips and walnuts, and combine in blender or food processor until smooth.

- Mix in the chips and nuts with a spoon to combine and pour into your greased pan.

- Bake at 350°F for 30 to 35 minutes until a toothpick comes out mostly clean. It won't be dry, but it shouldn't be gooey either.

- Cool on a cooling rack for about 20 minutes.

RAW BROWNIES

Delicious four-ingredient no-bake brownie recipe, gluten-free and vegan. An easy and healthy way to satisfy your sweet tooth!

Ingredients

2 cups organic walnuts

1 cup organic cocoa powder

2 cups organic dates, pitted

½ cup organic almonds, coarsely chopped

Method

- Add walnuts to the food processor until mixed to a powder. Combine the cocoa powder with the walnuts until mixed.

- Add the dates until the mixture becomes a thick dough. (Add a few at a time; you might not need the full 2 cups.) Make sure the dates are pitted before putting them into the Cuisinart food processor.

- Tip: Before you add the dates let them sit in hot water for about 10 minutes, so they become nice and soft.

- Place parchment paper inside an 8×8″ glass or metal dish. Add the brownie batter to the pan and sprinkle the almonds on top. Press the almonds into the batter and flatten in the pan until fully flat and even. Place in the fridge to harden for 15 to 20 minutes.

GANACHE

Ingredients

¼ cup organic coconut milk

4 ounces organic bittersweet or semisweet chocolate. (Try Lily's sugar-free stevia sweetened chocolate chips)

¼ teaspoon of salt

1 teaspoon on organic coconut oil

Method

- Combine all ingredients in a saucepan on low heat until the chocolate is melted. Add the melted chocolate to the cooled brownies; allow to cool for 10 minutes or until ganache is hardened.

- Pour yourself a glass of coconut milk and enjoy!

CHOCOLATE CHIP ALMOND BUTTER COOKIES

I am always looking for healthy alternatives to "old favorites." This is one of those recipes that tastes just as good and make you feel even better. Almonds are a healthy fat and plant-based protein that make a delicious base for these cookies!

Ingredients

1 cup organic almond butter

1 cup organic almond flour

1 cup Lily's sugar-free chocolate chips

1 flax egg

½ cup maple syrup, date syrup or granulated monk fruit

1 teaspoon baking soda

Method

- Combine all ingredients in a large bowl.
- Chill the dough in the fridge for at least 30 minutes, meanwhile preheat the oven to 350°F.
- Scoop dough onto a parchment-lined baking sheet and bake for 18 minutes

(Recipe adapted from Kale Junkie)

PUMPKIN CHOCOLATE CHIP
COOKIES (GLUTEN-FREE)

Fall is almost upon us and with the season comes all thoughts pumpkin. While fresh pumpkin may not be available all year long, canned or boxed organic pumpkin puree is always in your local grocery store and personally I always have some around for when I get a craving for these cookies.

I avoid refined flours and grains and that is why these cookies are a go-to favorite. They could not be easier to mix up, and you can be enjoying them within half an hour of having the idea that you are in the mood for cookies.

They are refined-sugar-free so will not get you craving anything bad. Feel free to substitute raisins, walnuts, currants or dried cherries for the chocolate. The almond flour provides healthy fat and protein and the result is a chewy, lightly sweet and satisfying cookie that makes you feel like you are cheating when it's truly a healthy treat.

They've been in my arsenal for so long I honestly don't remember how I came up with them, but likely it was some traditional white flour recipe that I "played with" until I could enjoy it without gluten, dairy or sugar.

Please let me know how you enjoy them.

Yield: 1 dozen cookies

Ingredients

1 ½ cups organic almond flour

¼ cup organic pumpkin puree, canned or from a box

¼ teaspoon baking soda

½ cup organic dark chocolate chips, dairy-free and sugar-free. (Try Lily's chocolate chips, or make your own using the recipe for *Dr Vikki's Homemade Sugar-Free Dark Chocolate* on my website, *www.RootCauseMedicalClinics*.com.) (Option: You can also substitute organic raisins or dried cherries if you are avoiding chocolate or sweeteners.)

1 large organic banana, very ripe and mashed well

¼ cup organic maple syrup

¼ cup organic coconut sugar, powdered date sugar, or granulated monk fruit sweetener

½ cup organic walnuts, chopped

1 teaspoon cinnamon

⅛ teaspoon nutmeg

⅛ teaspoon cloves

1 teaspoon pure vanilla extract

Method

- Heat oven to 350°F.
- Line a cookie sheet with parchment paper.
- Place all wet ingredients in a large bowl and whisk them thoroughly until well combined.
- Combine all dry ingredients together in a small bowl.
- Fold the dry mixture gradually into the wet ingredients until they are well combined. You can add a little more almond flour if the batter is thin. The mixture should be sticky and thick.

- Drop heaping teaspoons onto the prepared cookies sheet and press each gently to flatten them slightly.

- Place the cookies in the oven and bake for about 15 minutes or until they turn golden brown. Turn off the oven and let the cookies sit within the over for a couple of minutes.

- Remove from oven and slide parchment paper onto a wire rack and cool completely.

- Store in an airtight container in the refrigerator if there are any left!

PECAN PIE BARS

Gluten-free, dairy-free pecan pie bars – delicious without the sugar!

Pecan pie was always my favorite dessert at Thanksgiving. I know pumpkin and apple pies are universal favorites, but for me it was all about the pecan. Of course, the ingredients were sugar, brown sugar and corn syrup (more sugar!), compounded by butter and flour (gluten) in the crust. As someone who was sensitive to all of those ingredients, no wonder I felt so terrible after eating it. But I was unaware of my food sensitivities and all I knew was that a Thanksgiving without pecan pie was no Thanksgiving at all.

I well remember the fateful Thanksgiving where our large long-haired German Shepherd got up on the counter where the pie was cooling, pulled it on to the floor and licked it clean. All that remained was the crust.

We begged my mother to make a new one as it was still the night before Thanksgiving, but she refused. My siblings consoled themselves with the other available pies, but I was so disappointed.

Fast forward to gluten-free, dairy-free years and I have tried to adapt to new and healthier dietary habits while still offering a version of my favorite. When we added sugar-free to the roster of dietary exclusions, pecan pie seemed impossible. I have made a few attempts the past couple of years, but they were met with disappointment.

This year I decided to prepare early, and I was on a mission to find a "pie" (a bar in this case) that would be healthy, plant-based, gluten-free and sugar-free. Quite a tall order, but I found one, and it's delicious!

Much as my mother did, this recipe is best prepared the night before Thanksgiving or at least first thing in the morning Thanksgiving Day. It needs to set for about six hours. Just keep it away from any tall dogs!

Ingredients

"Shortbread" crust

⅓ cup organic coconut oil at room temperature (It's not melted, just at room temperature. It will be thick but soft, like room temperature butter.)

3 tablespoons organic maple syrup

¾ cup organic coconut flour, sifted. (If you don't have a sifter just put it through a fine sieve with a spoon. That will remove any lumps and add some air to it.)

a pinch of Himalayan sea salt

Pecan topping

2 flax eggs. To make flax eggs, take 2 tablespoons organic flax meal – or simply grind flax seeds in a coffee grinder – and add 5 tablespoon of warm water. Mix and place in refrigerator for about an hour or until well thickened. (You will have time for this while the crust is cooling.)

1 cup organic pecans, roughly chopped (don't make them too small because you want to "see" them and have a crunch to the topping.)

1 ½ tablespoons organic coconut oil

3 tablespoons organic maple syrup

½ cup organic date sugar or granulated monk fruit sweetener

¼ teaspoon Himalayan sea salt

Method

- Heat oven to 350°F.

- Line an 8×8" baking pan with parchment paper. Grease the sides of the pan with coconut oil.

- In a large bowl, beat the maple syrup and coconut oil together until creamy. Stir in the coconut flour and salt until it forms a dough.

- Press the dough evenly into the bottom of the pan and bake until the edges are a deep golden brown, and the middle is lightly golden, about 14 to 15 minutes. If the crust cracks, use the back of a spoon to press down on it and "seal" the crack.

- Let cool for 1 hour. You want the crust to be firm, so the topping does not make it soggy.

- Make the flax egg as described above and refrigerate; this will allow it to "gel".

- Place the pecans onto a cookie sheet in a single layer and bake them in the oven until they darken a bit and you can smell their aroma: about 8 to 10 minutes. Let cool, then roughly chop.

- Combine coconut oil, maple syrup, coconut sugar and salt in a large saucepan over medium heat and bring to a boil. Boil for one minute, stirring frequently and then remove from heat. Let it cool for 5 minutes at room temperature.

- Add the chilled flax eggs to the cooled mixture and combine well. Lastly, stir in the chopped pecans until they are well coated.

- Pour the topping over the crust, using a spoon to spread it out evenly. Press extra roughly chopped pecans lightly over the top so they lay flat and have the "look" that reminds you of the pecan pie of your youth!

- Bake until the filling looks set, about 20 minutes. Remove from the oven and let stand until it's no longer warm to the touch. Now place in the refrigerator for about 6 hours or overnight. This allows the bars to fully set.

- Slice and enjoy! For the holiday, consider preparing some coconut whipped cream as a topping.

- Please let me know how you enjoy this and remember you can prepare this dessert whenever you wish; you do not need to save it for Thanksgiving!

- (The source of the recipe is *foodfaithfitness.com*; I made some changes but the foundation of it was inspired by her and I thank her for the ingenuity in elevating a holiday favorite to a new level.)

NO-BAKE PUMPKIN PIE

I love pumpkin pie. But when I think about it I immediately get concerned about the crust. Crust is not the easiest undertaking at the best of times, but when you're talking about a gluten-free, dairy-free, sugar-free version, you're really setting yourself up for a challenge.

Is the crust flaky? Soggy? Too thick? Too thin?

This recipe takes ALL the stress out of crust making. It truly could not be simpler because it's raw. You just press it into a pie pan – four very healthy ingredients. It is sweet but has none of the "bad stuff".

The filling is equally delicious, creamy, full of pumpkin and spices, yet contains no dairy or sugar.

You will be surprised at the ease of this creamy pie and how well loved it will be. It is definitely a great addition to your dessert options, no matter what time of year it is.

Consider topping the pie with some coconut whipped cream when serving guests.

Please let us know how you enjoy it.

Ingredients

    1 cup dates, pit and stem removed

    1 cup organic raw cashews, unsalted

    ½ cup raw organic pecans or pecan pieces

    1 teaspoon organic cinnamon

    1 can (16 oz) organic pumpkin puree

½ cup organic coconut flour

½ cup organic coconut sugar or granulated monk fruit

2 teaspoons pumpkin pie spice

Method

- Soak the dates, cashews, and pecans in boiling water for 5 minutes.

- Drain the dates and nuts, then blend with the cinnamon seasoning in a food processor until smooth.

- Pour the mixture into a parchment-lined pie dish and flatten.

- Mix the pumpkin puree, coconut flour, coconut sugar and pumpkin pie spice in a bowl,

- stirring until well combined.

- Pour the pumpkin mixture over the crust layer, then store in the freezer until solid.

- Let pie defrost for about one hour prior to serving.

RAW CARROT CAKE WITH CREAMY CASHEW FROSTING

Do you love carrot cake? I do. What I remember most from childhood was that it was a dessert, it wasn't chocolate, it actually contained a vegetable, and I loved it!

Of course, I also remember the complete sugar "hangover" after eating it. How much sugar is involved in cream cheese frosting?! If memory serves it is an entire box of powdered sugar!

And yes, while the traditional version does certainly contain a vegetable, the poor carrot does not stand a chance amid all the sugar, dairy and gluten.

Could we create a version that had none of the negatives and bumped up the healthy options?

Oh yes; and this recipe really does it all. It's plant-based, gluten-, dairy- and sugar-free.

It is raw, making it ridiculously easy to make, but it's as satisfying as the traditional version with none of the excess sugar. In fact, there's zero refined sugar; the dates do the "sweet work" in the cake and some maple syrup handles the frosting.

The cake is quite filling; a small piece goes a long way.

You do not actually need to frost the cake if you don't want to. It is delicious, but the fat calories definitely rise from that, so it could be optional if you simply want to enjoy the cake.

As with all desserts, they are not for daily consumption, but honestly, frosting left off (or just cut in half), this is a dessert you could enjoy fairly often with no negative repercussions.

Ingredients

<u>For the base:</u>

    1 cup pitted organic dates

    1 cup shredded organic carrots

    1 cup organic walnuts

    ½ cup unsweetened organic coconut flakes

    ¼ cup organic coconut flour

    ¼ cup organic avocado oil

    1 teaspoon ground cinnamon

    ½ teaspoon ground ginger

    ¼ teaspoon nutmeg

    a pinch of pink Himalayan sea salt

<u>For the frosting:</u>

    2 cups organic raw cashews

    ¼ cup canned unsweetened coconut milk, shaken to mix well

    2 tablespoons organic avocado oil

    2 tablespoons filtered water

    3 tablespoons pure organic maple syrup

    3 teaspoons almond extract

    ¼ cup organic walnut pieces for topping

Method

- Set aside one regular loaf pan or two mini paper loaf pans (approximately 6″ L x 2.5″ W x 2″ H).

- Soak cashews in water for a minimum of 20 minutes, or boil for 10 minutes. Drain and set aside to cool.

- Soak dates in hot water for 15 minutes.

For the base:

- Mix dates in a food processor until a paste is formed. Evenly spread out the paste in a few chunks throughout the food processor.

- Add carrots, walnuts, coconut flakes, coconut flour, avocado oil, cinnamon, ginger, nutmeg, and pinch of sea salt to the date paste in the food processor. Combine until mixed together; adjust spices to taste.

- Divide in half and distribute contents into the two mini loaf pans; press evenly and store in freezer while making the frosting.

For the frosting:

- If you have not already, drain soaked cashews. In a blender, combine soaked cashews, coconut milk, oil, water, maple syrup and almond extract until smooth and creamy.

- Remove loaf from freezer and top evenly with frosting. Smooth the frosting with a mini spatula, or the back of a small spoon.

- Sprinkle the walnut pieces over the frosting and gently push into the frosting with your fingers to secure. Place loaf back into freezer for a minimum of 4 hours (or overnight).

- After the loaf has set, remove from the freezer, slice, and serve. Keep leftover carrot cake in an air-tight container in the freezer for up to 3 to 4 days.

(Recipe adapted from www.skinnykitlicious.com)

GINGER MOLASSES COOKIES

Servings: about thirty 3" cookies

Ingredients

- 2 cups gluten-free all-purpose flour (I used Bob's Red Mill Paleo baking flour to make it elimination diet-friendly)
- ½ teaspoon xanthan gum
- 1 teaspoon baking soda
- 1 teaspoon baking powder
- 1 ½ teaspoons ground ginger
- 1 teaspoon ground cinnamon
- ½ teaspoon ground nutmeg
- ½ teaspoon ground cloves
- ½ cup vegan butter (I used Earth Balance soy-free vegan butter to make it elimination diet-friendly)
- ¾ cup coconut sugar, plus additional sugar for rolling
- ½ cup blackstrap molasses
- 1 tablespoon water

Method

- Preheat the oven to 350°F.
- Line a large baking sheet with parchment paper, or Silpat.
- In a medium mixing bowl, whisk flour, xanthan gum, baking soda, baking powder, ginger, cinnamon, nutmeg, and cloves. Set aside.

- Using a stand or hand mixer, beat the vegan butter, coconut sugar, molasses, and water until well combined (creamed). Slowly beat in the flour mixture little by little.

- Scoop about 1 rounded tablespoon of dough at a time and roll the domed part of each scoop in the additional coconut sugar. Place the scoops onto the prepared baking sheet, making sure the sugar-topped side is facing up.

- Bake for 10 to 12 minutes, rotating halfway.

- Let cool on pan for 5 minutes. Enjoy!

SPICED APPLESAUCE CAKE

What is not to love when you think of spice cake? The combination of cinnamon, nutmeg and ginger just screams "Fall" and right through the holidays. Honestly, if you enjoy these flavors there is really no season that's a wrong one to enjoy them.

Applesauce has always been a "secret" ingredient in baking that provides an effortless moistness and this cake is definitely moist. When you pair the ease of adding some pre-made applesauce with a flour blend from Bob's Red Mill, this is a very simple recipe.

I was thrilled when Bob's Red Mill came out with their paleo baking flour mix. It contains almond flour, coconut flour, arrowroot and tapioca starch, and that's it! Pretty clean, grain-free and all pre-mixed, making it a very nice flour mix to have around.

Personally, I need to stay away from refined grain-based flours, but this mix is free from all grains. The root starches make it high in fiber, a very good thing, so despite the coconut sugar, you should not find yourself craving sugar after this dessert.

The frosting is not required. It has coconut butter, which is high in saturated fat, but if you only use this for special occasions then it's totally fine.

Please let me know how you enjoy it and if you come up with any variations you enjoy.

Ingredients

- 2 ¼ cups Bob's Red Mill Paleo gluten-free baking flour (a blend of nut flours and root starches)
- 1 teaspoon xanthan gum

2 teaspoons baking soda

1 teaspoon Himalayan sea salt

1 ½ teaspoons ground organic cinnamon

½ teaspoon ground organic nutmeg

½ teaspoon ground organic ginger

2 cups unsweetened organic applesauce

1 cup organic coconut sugar, or date sugar, or granulated monk fruit

½ cup organic avocado oil

¼ cup organic apple cider vinegar

1 tablespoon pure organic vanilla extract

½ cup unsweetened organic raisins (or currants), tossed in ½ tablespoon of Bob's Red Mill Paleo baking flour

½ cup chopped organic walnuts, tossed in ½ tablespoon of Bob's Red Mill Paleo baking flour

Frosting

2 to 3 tablespoons organic coconut butter, melted

1 tablespoon granulated sweetener of choice (consider date sugar or coconut sugar)

Organic dairy-free milk to thin out (we used almond milk)

Method

- Preheat the oven to 350°F. Lightly grease a 9×9 baking pan.

- In a large bowl, whisk together flour, xanthan gum, baking soda, salt, cinnamon, nutmeg, and ginger.

- In a separate bowl, whisk together applesauce, coconut sugar, oil, vinegar, and vanilla. Pour the wet mixture into the dry mixture and whisk until just combined. Do not overmix.

- Gently fold in flour-coated raisins and walnuts. Fill the prepared pan evenly with batter.

- Bake for 60 minutes – rotate the cake the cake halfway through baking time – then check if fully cooked. Depending on your oven, it may take 15 more minutes. Cook until a toothpick inserted in the center of the cake comes out dry with a few crumbs clinging to it.

- Let the cake cool completely.

- Mix the frosting in bowl and cool in refrigerator to thicken. Drizzle frosting.

OATMEAL NUT CHOCOLATE BARS

These bars are delicious, they contain no gluten, dairy or sugar, are fully plant-based, and oh so easy to make. What I like about them is they transport well to school or work or picnic. It's a one-bowl affair, making clean-up a breeze. Plus they're raw, so zero cooking time.

These are a spin-off of our Best Energy Bites, which is also in this chapter, but their flatter shape might make them easier to transport.

Start with organic, certified gluten-free oats and then choose your favorite nut (remember the best anti-cancer nuts are raw, organic walnuts, pecans and the "non-nut" peanut). Did you know that daily nut eaters had fewer deaths from heart disease and cancer as opposed to those not consuming nuts? You do not need a lot of nuts to retain this health benefit. A little goes a long way in preventing disease.

I like to lightly toast my nuts to bring out their flavor profile. It just takes a few minutes in a dry sauté pan on the stovetop.

Next choose the nut butter of your choice (almond, peanut, etc.) Make sure it is organic and has no additional ingredients beyond the nuts and perhaps a little salt.

For the chocolate component you can make my homemade sugar-free dark chocolate recipe or buy a pure cacao bar or pieces with no added sugar. The latter is more bitter, but it is still good. My recipe uses natural date sweetener, so it has some sweetness but it is mild.

If you do not like chocolate you can easily substitute raisins, dried cranberries or whatever suits you; just ensure they're organic with no added sugar.

I really prefer you use date syrup over any other sweetener because it is truly the only whole food sweetener out there other than stevia (which wouldn't work in this recipe).

Please let me know how you enjoy these and any fun combinations you and your family enjoy!

Servings: 10 bars

Ingredients

- 1 ¾ cups old-fashioned oats (break them up a bit in a blender or food processor)
- 1 ⅓ cups chopped organic walnuts, pecans, or almonds (lightly toasted)
- ⅔ cup chopped pure sugar-free dark chocolate (Use our recipe for homemade sugar-free dark chocolate or just buy a pure cacao bar with no sugar.) (Option: Use raisins or dried cranberries instead of the chocolate.)
- ¼ teaspoon Himalayan sea salt
- 1 cup creamy organic peanut butter or almond butter
- scant ½ cup organic date syrup
- 1 ½ teaspoons vanilla extract
- Optional: 1 teaspoon ground cinnamon (my family likes it better without)

Method

- Line an 8×9″ square Pyrex with parchment paper.
- In a mixing bowl, combine the broken-up oats, chopped toasted nuts, chocolate, cinnamon (if you're using it) and salt. Whisk to combine.

- Measure out the nut butter in a 2-cup liquid measuring cup and add the scant ½ cup date syrup and vanilla on top. Whisk until blended.

- Pour the liquid ingredients onto the dry ingredients and use a large spoon (or your hands!) to combine it all, ensuring all the oats are coated and not dry.

- Transfer the mixture to your glass pan and press down to distribute it evenly, pressing firmly to compact it. (You can use your hands or something flat, like the bottom of a glass.)

- Refrigerate for at least one hour, cut into bars and enjoy.

- You can wrap bars in plastic or parchment paper for easy transport or keep covered in the fridge. You can even freeze them, although ours never last that long!

CHOCOLATE PEANUT BUTTER RICE CRISPY TREATS

Who has never had a Rice Krispie Treat? Not many Americans I would imagine. They are easy to make, loaded with sugar and butter (unfortunately), but you have to admit, adding chocolate on top was definitely a good idea.

Recently we were traveling, and a coffee shop had them. The serving was HUGE. I don't often crave dessert, but this just looked good. It was probably the generous amount of chocolate on top!

I looked at my daughter and suggested we try and make them without sugar, dairy, high fructose corn syrup, etc, etc.

Not surprisingly, I was not the first to think of it. There were several recipes online that we looked over, and then created our own version.

I like the fact that our recipe has zero sugar, dairy or gluten, and uses organic brown rice crispies and organic peanut butter. They are delicious, yet very easy to make. We hope you enjoy them!

Ingredients

Rice crispy base

- ¾ cup creamy organic sugar-free peanut butter (Option: almond butter or SunButter)
- ⅓ cup raw honey
- ¼ teaspoon sea salt
- ½ teaspoon pure vanilla extract
- 3 cups crispy organic brown rice cereal

Chocolate peanut butter topping

- 1 ½ cups (6 ounces) Lily's stevia-sweetened dark chocolate, either the bar or the chips
- 1 ½ tablespoons creamy organic no sugar peanut butter

Method

Rice crispy base

- Line an 8×8" or 9×9" square glass baking pan with parchment paper. Lightly grease with avocado oil and set aside.
- On the stovetop over medium-low heat, melt together the honey and peanut butter, stirring until combined (be very careful to not overheat).
- Remove from heat and stir in the sea salt and vanilla extract until combined.
- Add the crispy rice cereal to a large clean & dry mixing bowl.
- Pour peanut butter mixture on top of the cereal and stir until completely combined.
- Pour mixture into the prepared baking pan. Use a greased spatula to spread it until the top is even and smooth.

Chocolate peanut butter topping

- Melt the chocolate and peanut butter together on the stovetop over medium-low heat, stirring until just combined. Be careful to not overheat.

<u>Assembly</u>

- Pour the topping over the rice crispy treat base, using a spatula to spread it evenly and smoothly.

- Place treats in the refrigerator for 60 minutes (or in the freezer for a shorter chill time).

- Remove 5 to 10 minutes before serving to let them warm up slightly before cutting, otherwise the chocolate will crack.

- Serve at room temperature.

- Store in an airtight container in the refrigerator.

VEGAN BERRY CRISP

Crisps are delicious and satisfying and can adapt to any season depending on the fruit you choose to use. This recipe is berry-inspired which makes it very healthy, considering berries are one of the best fruits to eat.

> **Note:** If you use strawberries, they must be organic since strawberries are on the "Dirty Dozen" list of the most pesticide-laden fruits. Pesticides aside, strawberries are best when mixed with other berries since they have a high-water content. You do not want soupy crisp.

You may use varying combinations of berries. You can even add in fresh peaches or any fruits in season.

If you are feeling festive, consider topping it with coconut whipped cream or a non-dairy ice cream with no sugar. Yes, there are some pretty delicious sugar-free, dairy-free ice creams on the market.

The crisp is best served warm.

We hope you will love this recipe as much as we do!

Ingredients

Filling:

- 7 to 8 cups mixed organic berries (strawberries, raspberries, blueberries, and/or blackberries)

- 3 tablespoons organic maple syrup

- 2 tablespoons arrowroot starch (optional: substitute cornstarch or gluten-free flour)

1 tablespoon organic lemon juice

<u>Crisp:</u>

1 cup organic almond flour (or almond meal)

⅔ cup shredded or desiccated coconut

1 cup roughly chopped organic walnuts, pecans (or other nut of choice)

½ cup organic coconut sugar

½ teaspoon sea salt

4 tablespoons organic refined coconut oil or vegan butter

Optional: 2 tablespoons maple syrup

Method

- Preheat oven to 350°F.

- Add fruit to a 9×13″ glass dish. Top the fruit with maple syrup, arrowroot, and lemon juice; toss to combine.

- In a large mixing bowl, combine the almond flour, coconut, pecans (or whatever nut you are using), coconut sugar, and salt. Stir to combine.

- Add coconut oil (or vegan butter) and mix again (with a spoon or your hands) until it is evenly distributed.

- It is good to taste at this point – see if it's sweet enough for you. If not, add either more coconut sugar or a little maple syrup, about 2 tablespoons.

- Spread the crisp topping evenly over the fruit. Bake uncovered on the center oven rack for 40 to 45 minutes or until the fruit is bubbling and the top is golden brown.

- Let cool 10 minutes before serving. Store leftovers covered in the refrigerator up to 4 days.

- (Grateful acknowledgement to Oh She Glows and the Minimalist Baker for inspiration of this recipe.)

CHOCOLATE CHUNK BANANA BREAD

Chocolatey banana bread with walnuts

Does everyone love banana bread? Based on the tens of millions of hits on a Google search, apparently yes. It's a favorite because it is moist, chocolatey, crunchy with nuts, and can be enjoyed for a snack, breakfast and dessert. So adaptable!

The traditional recipe is full of gluten, sugar, milk, eggs and is basically completely unhealthy. Taking on the challenge of creating a healthy version was fun and I think you will enjoy it.

This recipe is free of most allergens and very easy to make.

If you are avoiding nuts, you can just leave them out, or add sunflower or pumpkin seeds. If you are avoiding oats you can substitute quinoa flakes.

Enjoy the recipe for special occasions and wow your friends and family who won't believe you made it from scratch. It is that good!

Let me know how you enjoy it and any substitutions you try.

You will need a 9×5″ loaf pan. (I prefer glass.)

Ingredients

- 1 ⅓ cups mashed very ripe banana (about 4 medium or 3 large)
- 2 tablespoons ground organic flaxseed
- ⅓ cup organic unsweetened plant-based milk, such as almond milk

⅓ cup organic refined coconut oil, melted (or use unrefined if you enjoy the flavor of coconut)

2 tablespoons pure organic maple syrup, date syrup or granulated monk fruit

2 teaspoons pure vanilla extract

Dry ingredients

¼ cup plus 2 tablespoons organic coconut sugar or date sugar

½ cup organic gluten-free rolled oats

1 teaspoon baking soda

½ teaspoon baking powder

½ teaspoon Himalayan sea salt

1 ½ cups Bob's Red Mill all-purpose gluten-free flour mix

¾ cup organic chopped walnuts, divided

¼ cup bittersweet chocolate, roughly chopped (high quality, dairy-free and preferably sugar-free, such as Lily's stevia-sweetened chocolate chips.)

Method

- Preheat the oven to 350°F. Lightly grease a 9×5″ loaf pan with coconut oil.

- In a large bowl, mash the banana well.

- Add the remaining wet ingredients (almond milk, melted oil, maple syrup, and vanilla) into the banana and mix until combined.

- Stir the dry ingredients (ground flax, coconut sugar, oats, baking soda, baking powder, salt, and flour) into the wet mixture, one by one, in the order listed. Do not overmix. As soon as all the ingredients are combined, stop.

- Lastly add the walnuts (½ cup) and chocolate.

- Spoon the dough into the loaf pan and spread it evenly. Add the remaining ¼ cup of walnuts to the top of the dough, gently pressing them into the dough.

- Bake the loaf, uncovered, for 45 to 50 minutes until lightly golden and firm on top. The top of the loaf should slowly spring back when you press on it.

- Set the loaf pan on a cooling rack for 20 minutes; allow to cool completely.

- Loosen with a knife and remove it from the pan, placing it again onto the cooling rack. It is hard to wait, I know!

- The loaf will keep in the fridge tightly wrapped for 3 to 4 days, or it can be frozen for 4 to 5 weeks.

ACKNOWLEDGMENTS

We would like to acknowledge the innovators and bright minds in this world who refuse to be told they cannot, and instead move only towards what can be and should be, for the greater good of all.

Our planet is not always kind to the original thinker, the one who pushes back against what "is" and refuses to be a part of what is deemed "acceptable" by the masses.

It is not a comfortable role to play because criticism and derision abounds. Yet for those intrepid few who have lofty goals that truly benefit the greatest number of individuals, nothing will veer them off their path, and nothing should.

We acknowledge your courage and determination and thank you for all that you do to make our world a better, safer, and healthier place.

The staff of Root Cause Medical Clinics is a very special group of individuals. We thank you for joining us on our mission to bring sane and effective healthcare to our planet. You are all wonderful, amazingly dedicated, and we consider you family.

Dr Rupa Chakravarty, our Doctor of Physical Therapy, deserves to be acknowledged for the innovative work she is bringing to Hiatal Hernia Syndrome. Her discoveries of precise influences of the nervous system on the condition were not yet sufficiently complete to include in this book, but hopefully in the not-too-distant future, the work she is doing with patients at Root Cause will be codified.

Our CEO, Nandita Mahadevan, is a very special member of our team who cannot be thanked enough for all that she contributes. A friend, consigliere, and visionary, she is truly the best of the best.

We would like to thank our friend and mentor, Lisa Everett Andersen, a brilliant Clinical Pharmacist, and author of the acclaimed text *Learning to Thrive in a Toxic World*. Lisa is a selfless healer and we feel blessed to have her in our lives.

A special thank you to our friend and advisor Kay Daly, an incredible woman who has seemed to live nine lives, all unique and exciting, while maintaining a love for her fellow man that few embody. You are loved.

And finally, we would like to thank our amazing children for all their wonderful contributions to this world. We could not be more proud nor impressed with the wonderful people you are. The mutual goals we share while having fun and supporting each other is truly special. Let the adventure continue!

INDEX

ADDITIONAL RESEARCH PAPERS

1. Yoshida N. Inflammation and oxidative stress in gastroesophageal reflux disease. *J Clin Biochem Nutr.* 2007;40(1):13-23.

2. Surjushe A, Vasani R, Saple D. Aloe vera: a short review. *Indian J Dermatol.* 2008;53(4):163-166.

3. Savarino E, de Bortoli N, Zentilin P, et al. Alginate controls heartburn in patients with erosive and nonerosive reflux disease. *World J Gastroenterol.* 2012;18(32):4371-4378.

4. Kumari CS, Prasad CVN, Ramulu JS. Determination of in-vitro and in-vivo activities of Aloe vera L. against H. pylori. *Int J Pharma Bio Sci.* 2010;1(2):1-8.

5. Cellini L, Di Bartolomeo S, Di Campli E, Genovese S, Locatelli M, Di Giulio M. In vitro activity of Aloe vera inner gel against Helicobacter pylori strains. *Lett Appl Microbiol.* 2014;59(1):43-48.

6. Asadi-Shahmirzadi A, Mozaffari S, Sanei Y, et al. Benefit of Aloe vera and Matricaria recutita mixture in rat irritable bowel syndrome: combination of antioxidant and spasmolytic effects [published online ahead of print December 21, 2012]. *Chin J Integr Med.* doi:*10.1007/s11655-012-1027-9.*

7. Langmead L, Feakins RM, Goldthorpe S, et al. Randomized, double-blind, placebo-controlled trial of oral aloe vera gel for active ulcerative colitis. *Aliment Pharmacol Ther.* 2004;19(7):739-747.

8. Korkina L, Suprun M, Petrova A, Mikhal'chik E, Luci A, De Luca C. The protective and healing effects of a natural antioxidant formulation based on ubiquinol and Aloe vera against dextran sulfate-induced ulcerative colitis in rats. *Biofactors.* 2003;18(1-4):255-264.

9. Yusuf S, Agunu A, Diana M. The effect of Aloe vera A. Berger (Liliaceae) on gastric acid secretion and acute gastric mucosal injury in rats. *J Ethnopharmacol.* 2004;93(1):33-37.

10. Borra SK, Lagisetty RK, Mallela GR. Anti-ulcer effect of Aloe vera in non-steroidal anti-inflammatory drug induced peptic ulcers in rats. *Afr J Pharm Pharmacol.* 2011;5:1867–1871.

11. Yu EW, Bauer SR, Bain PA, Bauer DC. Proton pump inhibitors and risk of fractures: a meta-analysis of 11 international studies. *Am J Med.* 2011;124(6):519-526.

12. Khalili H, Huang ES, Jacobson BC, Camargo CA, Feskanich D, Chan AT. Use of proton pump inhibitors and risk of hip fracture in relation to dietary and lifestyle factors: a prospective cohort study. *BMJ.* 2012;344:e372.

13. Gomm W, von Holt K, Thomé F, et al. Association of proton pump inhibitors with risk of dementia: a pharmacoepidemiological claims data analysis. *JAMA Neurol.* 2016;73(4):410-416.

14. Seto CT, Jeraldo P, Orenstein R, Chia N, DiBaise JK. Prolonged use of a proton pump inhibitor reduces microbial diversity: implications for Clostridium difficile susceptibility. *Microbiome.* 2014;2:42.

15. Shah NH, LePendu P, Bauer-Mehren A, et al. Proton pump inhibitor usage and the risk of myocardial infarction in the general population. *PLoS One.* 2015;10(6):e0124653.

16. Lazarus B, Chen Y, Wilson FP, et al. Proton pump inhibitor use and the risk of chronic kidney disease. *JAMA Intern Med.* 2016;176(2):238-246.

17. Yepuri G, Sukhovershin R, Nazari-Shafti TZ, Petrascheck M, Ghebre YT, Cooke JP. Proton pump inhibitors accelerate endothelial senescence. *Circ Res.* 2016;118(12);e36-42.

18. Thorens J, Froehlich F, Schwizer W, et al. Bacterial overgrowth during treatment with omeprazole compared with cimetidine: a prospective randomised double blind study. *Gut.* 1996;39(1):54-59.

19. Fullarton GM, McLauchlan G, Macdonald A, Crean GP, McColl KE. Rebound nocturnal hypersecretion after four weeks treatment with an H2 receptor antagonist. *Gut.* 1989;30(4):449-454.

20. Valuck RJ, Ruscin JM. A case-control study on adverse effects: H2 blocker or proton pump inhibitor use and risk of vitamin B12 deficiency in older adults. *J Clin Epidemiol.* 2004;57(4):422-428.

21. Penston J, Wormsley KG. Adverse reactions and interactions with H2-receptor antagonists. *Med Toxicol.* 1986;1(3):192-216.

22. Festi D, Scaioli E, Baldi F, et al. Body weight, lifestyle, dietary habits and gastroesophageal reflux disease. *World J Gastroenterol.* 2009;15(14):1690-1701.

23. Song JH, Chung SJ, Lee JH, et al. Relationship between gastroesophageal reflux symptoms and dietary factors in Korea. *J Neurogastroenterol Motil.* 2011;17(1):54-60.

24. Austin GL, Thiny MT, Westman EC, Yancy WS Jr, Shaheen NJ. A very low-carbohydrate diet improves gastroesophageal reflux and its symptoms. *Dig Dis Sci.* 2006;51(8):1307-1312.

25. Singh M, Lee J, Gupta N, et al. Weight loss can lead to resolution of gastroesophageal reflux disease symptoms: a prospective intervention trial. Obesity (Silver Spring). 2013;21(2):284-290.

26. Sun J. D-Limonene: safety and clinical applications. *Altern Med Rev.* 2007;12(3):259-264.

27. Kandil TS, Mousa AA, El-Gendy AA, Abbas AM. The potential therapeutic effect of melatonin in gastro-esophageal reflux disease. *BMC Gastroenterol.* 2010;10:7.

28. Melzer J, Rosch W, Reichling J, Brignoli R, Saller R. Meta-analysis: phytotherapy of functional dyspepsia with the herbal drug preparation STW 5 (Iberogast). *Aliment Pharmacol Ther.* 2004;20(11-12):1279-1287.

29. Meletis CD, Zabriskie N. Natural approaches for gastroesophageal reflux disease and related disorders. *Altern Complement Ther.* 2007;13(2):64-70.

30. Sandberg-Lewis S. Proton pump inhibitors-a risky experiment? *Townsend Letter for Doctors and Patients. http://www.townsendletter. com/FebMarch2011/protonpump0211.html.* Published February, 2011. Accessed July 8, 2016.

31. Patrick L. Gastroesophageal reflux disease (GERD): a review of conventional and alternative treatments. *Altern Med Rev.* 2011;16(2):116-133.

CPSIA information can be obtained
at www.ICGtesting.com
Printed in the USA
LVHW051047261021
701572LV00011B/214

9 780982 271148